LOW SODIUM MEDITERRANEAN DIET COOKBOOK

A Dietary Guide with 50 Delicious Low Salt Recipes, Meal Plan, and Lifestyle Tips to Lower Blood Pressure and Improve Heart Health

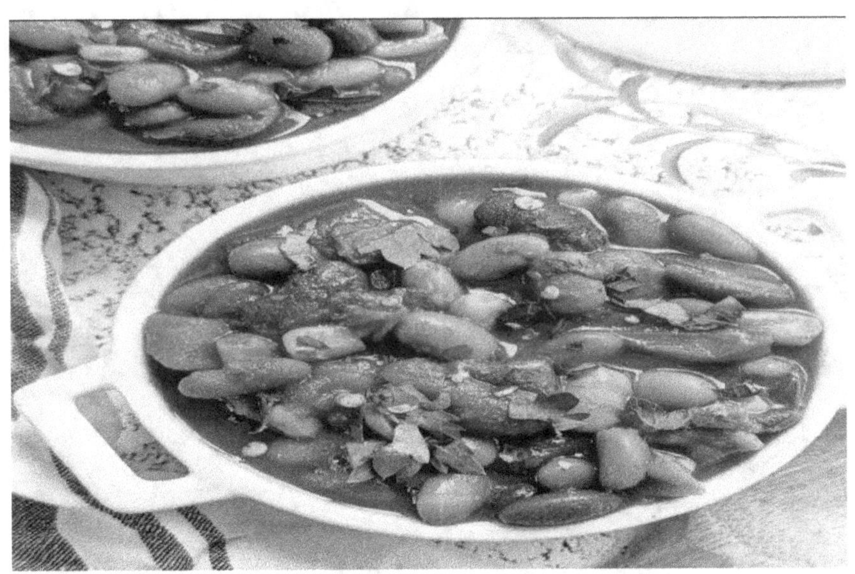

DR. COLE HULL

COPYRIGHT

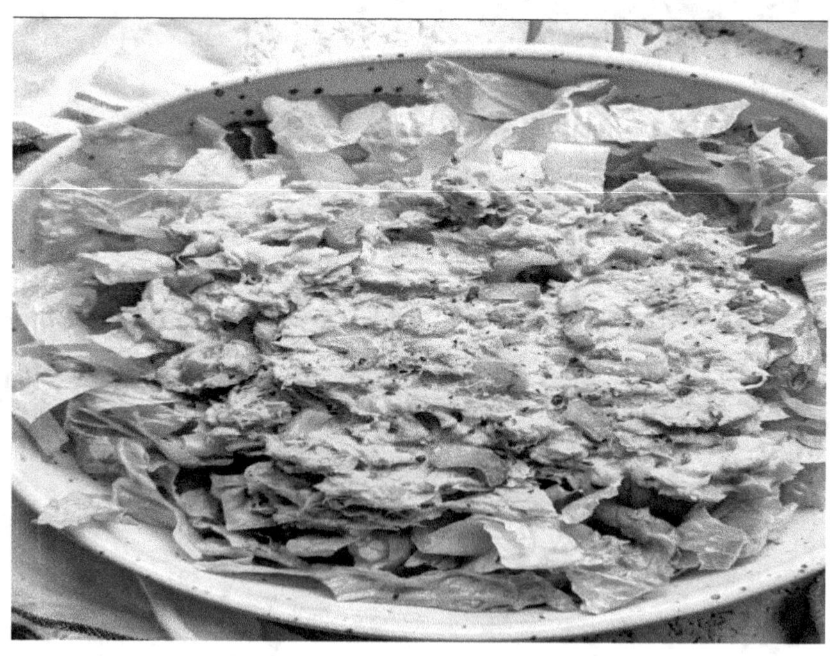

TABLE OF CONTENT

1. INTRODUCTION

The low sodium Mediterranean diet is a variation of the traditional Mediterranean diet that emphasizes reducing sodium intake. The Mediterranean diet is known for its heart-healthy benefits and is characterized by a high consumption of fruits, vegetables, whole grains, legumes, nuts, and olive oil, moderate consumption of fish and poultry, and low consumption of red meat and sweets. It also includes a moderate intake of wine, typically with meals.

In a low sodium Mediterranean diet, the focus is on limiting foods that are high in sodium, such as processed and canned foods, salty snacks, and cured meats, while still following the principles of the Mediterranean diet. This approach is particularly beneficial for individuals with hypertension or cardiovascular disease, as reducing sodium intake can help lower blood pressure and improve heart health.

The low sodium Mediterranean diet promotes the use of herbs and spices for flavoring instead of salt, and encourages the consumption of fresh, whole foods to naturally keep sodium levels low. It is a balanced and nutritious diet that can support overall health and well-being.

Overview of the Low Sodium Mediterranean Diet

The Mediterranean diet is celebrated for its numerous health benefits, including improved heart health, weight management, and reduced risk of chronic diseases. It is a dietary pattern inspired by the traditional eating habits of the countries bordering the Mediterranean Sea, such as Italy, Greece, and Spain. The diet emphasizes whole foods, including fruits, vegetables, whole grains, legumes, nuts, seeds, and olive oil, as the primary source of fat. It also includes moderate amounts of fish, poultry, and dairy, with limited intake of red meat and sweets.

The low sodium Mediterranean diet takes the core principles of the traditional Mediterranean diet and modifies them to further support cardiovascular health by reducing sodium intake. This adaptation is particularly beneficial for individuals with hypertension, heart disease, or those simply looking to lower their sodium consumption for overall wellness. By focusing on fresh, unprocessed foods and using herbs and spices for flavoring instead of salt, the low sodium Mediterranean diet offers a delicious and healthful way to eat.

Benefits of Reducing Sodium Intake

The benefits of reducing sodium intake are well-documented and can have a significant impact on overall health, particularly for those with or at risk of hypertension and cardiovascular diseases. Here are some key benefits:

1. Lower Blood Pressure: High sodium intake is a major contributor to elevated blood pressure. By reducing sodium in your diet, you can help lower your blood pressure levels, reducing the strain on your heart and arteries.

2. Reduced Risk of Heart Disease: Lowering sodium intake is associated with a decreased risk of developing heart disease. By following a low sodium diet, you can help keep your heart healthy and strong.

3. Improved Heart Health: A diet low in sodium can improve the health of your heart by reducing the risk of stroke, heart failure, and other cardiovascular conditions.

4. Better Kidney Function: Excessive sodium can put a strain on your kidneys, which are responsible for filtering and removing waste from your body. A low sodium diet can support better kidney function and health.

5. Prevention of Fluid Retention: High sodium levels can cause your body to retain excess fluid, leading to swelling and discomfort. Reducing sodium intake can help prevent fluid retention and its associated symptoms.

6. Weight Management: While sodium itself doesn't cause weight gain, a diet high in processed and high-sodium foods can contribute to weight gain. By choosing low sodium, whole foods, you can support a healthy weight.

7. Enhanced Taste Sensitivity: Over time, reducing your sodium intake can help recalibrate your taste buds, making you more sensitive to the natural flavors of food. This can enhance your overall eating experience and enjoyment of food.

Incorporating a low sodium Mediterranean diet into your lifestyle can help you reap these benefits while enjoying a diverse and delicious array of foods. In the next section, we'll explore the Mediterranean lifestyle and how it complements a low sodium diet.

The Mediterranean Lifestyle

The Mediterranean lifestyle is about more than just food; it's a holistic approach to living that emphasizes balance, well-being, and the enjoyment of life. Here are some key aspects of the Mediterranean lifestyle that complement a low sodium diet:

1. Enjoying Meals with Others: Sharing meals with family and friends is a central part of the Mediterranean lifestyle. It's an opportunity to connect, relax, and savor the experience of eating.

2. Mindful Eating: The Mediterranean lifestyle encourages mindfulness in eating, which means paying attention to the flavors, textures, and aromas of your food, as well as listening to your body's hunger and fullness cues.

3. Physical Activity: Regular physical activity is an integral part of the Mediterranean lifestyle. Whether it's walking, swimming, or dancing, find activities that you enjoy and make them a part of your daily routine.

4. Stress Management: Managing stress is important for overall health. The Mediterranean lifestyle encourages practices such as meditation, spending time in nature, and engaging in hobbies to help reduce stress.

5. *Moderation:* The Mediterranean lifestyle is about balance and moderation. It's not about strict rules or deprivation but about making mindful choices that support your health and well-being.

By embracing the Mediterranean lifestyle, you can enhance the benefits of a low sodium diet and enjoy a healthier, more balanced life. In the following chapters, we'll provide you with delicious recipes, practical tips, and inspiration to help you live the low sodium Mediterranean lifestyle to the fullest.

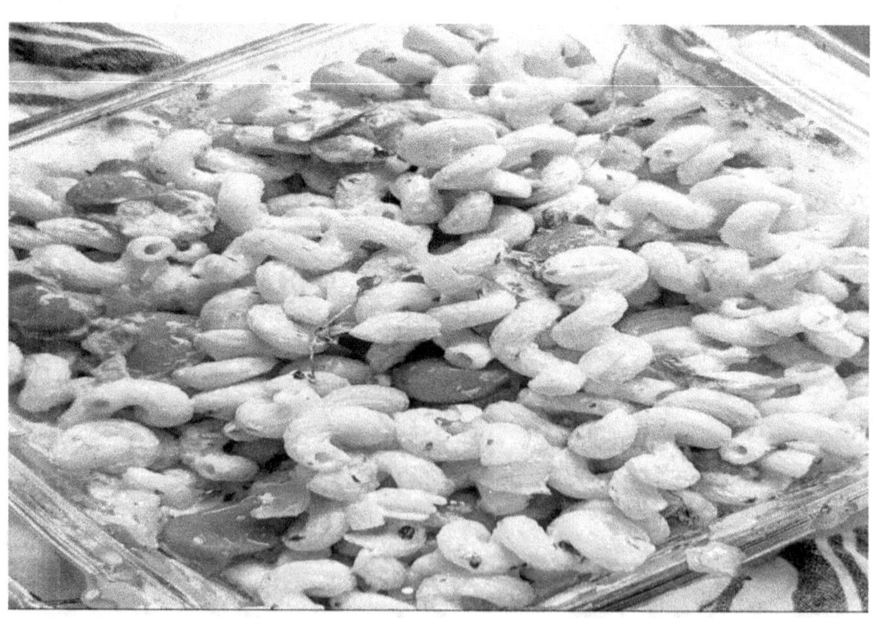

2. UNDERSTANDING SODIUM

Sodium is a crucial mineral in our diet, playing a vital role in various bodily functions. However, it's essential to understand its impact on our health to make informed dietary choices, especially when following a low sodium Mediterranean diet.

The Role of Sodium in the Body

Sodium is an electrolyte that helps maintain fluid balance in the body, supports nerve function, and assists in muscle contraction. It is essential for maintaining blood pressure and volume and plays a role in the absorption of other nutrients, such as glucose and amino acids. Sodium is naturally present in many foods and is commonly added in the form of table salt (sodium chloride).

In the right amounts, sodium is beneficial and necessary for health. However, the body requires only a small amount of sodium to function properly. The kidneys regulate sodium levels in the body, excreting any excess through urine. When the balance of sodium is disrupted, it can lead to health issues.

The Risks of High Sodium Intake

While sodium is essential for health, consuming too much can lead to several health problems. The most well-known risk associated with high sodium intake is hypertension, or high blood pressure. High blood pressure increases the risk of heart disease, stroke, and kidney disease.

Excessive sodium intake can also lead to fluid retention, causing swelling in the legs, feet, and hands. This can be particularly problematic for individuals with heart failure or kidney disease.

In addition to these risks, high sodium intake has been linked to other health issues, such as osteoporosis, stomach cancer, and exacerbation of asthma symptoms. It's important to note that the risks associated with high sodium intake are not limited to those with existing health conditions; even healthy individuals can benefit from reducing their sodium intake to prevent future health problems.

Reducing sodium intake can lower blood pressure, reduce the risk of cardiovascular disease, and improve overall health. This is where the low sodium Mediterranean diet comes into play, offering a delicious and healthful way to enjoy food while keeping sodium intake in check.

How to Identify High Sodium Foods

When following a low sodium Mediterranean diet, it's crucial to know how to identify high sodium foods to make informed choices. Here are some tips to help you recognize and avoid foods that are high in sodium:

1. Read Nutrition Labels: Check the sodium content on the nutrition facts label of packaged foods. Look for items with less than 140 milligrams of sodium per serving, which are considered low sodium. Be mindful of the serving size, as consuming multiple servings can quickly add up to a high sodium intake.

2. Watch Out for Processed Foods: Processed and packaged foods, such as canned soups, frozen dinners, snack foods, and deli meats, are often high in sodium. Opt for fresh or minimally processed alternatives whenever possible.

3. Be Cautious with Condiments: Condiments like soy sauce, ketchup, salad dressings, and marinades can be high in sodium. Look for low sodium versions or use herbs and spices to flavor your food instead.

4. Limit Fast Food and Restaurant Meals: Fast food and restaurant dishes are often high in sodium. When dining out, ask for your meal to be prepared with less salt, and choose dishes that are grilled, baked, or steamed rather than fried.

5. Choose Fresh or Frozen Vegetables: Canned vegetables can be high in sodium due to added salt. Opt for fresh or frozen vegetables, which are usually lower in sodium and just as nutritious.

6. Rinse Canned Foods: If you do use canned foods, such as beans or tuna, rinse them under water to remove some of the sodium.

7. Cook from Scratch: Cooking meals at home allows you to control the amount of sodium in your dishes. Use fresh ingredients and season your food with herbs, spices, lemon juice, or vinegar instead of salt.

By becoming adept at identifying high sodium foods and making smarter choices, you can successfully follow a low sodium Mediterranean diet and enjoy the numerous health benefits it offers. In the next section, we'll delve into the essentials of the low sodium Mediterranean diet, providing you with the knowledge and tools to embrace this heart-healthy way of eating.

3. THE ESSENTIALS OF THE LOW SODIUM MEDITERRANEAN DIET

The low sodium Mediterranean diet is a heart-healthy eating plan that combines the traditional Mediterranean diet's principles with a focus on reducing sodium intake. This section will explore the key components and foods that make up this diet, the importance of fresh and whole foods, and how to use herbs and spices for flavor without relying on salt.

Key Components and Foods

The low sodium Mediterranean diet is centered around a variety of nutrient-dense, whole foods that provide a plethora of health benefits. Here are the key components and foods that form the foundation of this diet:

1. Fruits and Vegetables: These are the cornerstone of the low sodium Mediterranean diet. Aim to fill half your plate with a colorful array of fruits and vegetables at each meal. They are low in sodium and rich in vitamins, minerals, antioxidants, and fiber.

2. *Whole Grains:* Opt for whole grains like quinoa, brown rice, barley, oats, and whole wheat pasta. These provide essential nutrients and fiber, which can help regulate blood pressure and support heart health.

3. *Legumes:* Beans, lentils, and chickpeas are excellent protein sources and are rich in fiber, which can help lower cholesterol and blood pressure.

4. *Nuts and Seeds:* Almonds, walnuts, flaxseeds, and chia seeds are packed with healthy fats, protein, and fiber. Just be sure to choose unsalted varieties to keep sodium intake in check.

5. *Healthy Fats:* Olive oil is the primary source of added fat in the low sodium Mediterranean diet. It's rich in monounsaturated fats, which can help reduce bad cholesterol levels and lower the risk of heart disease.

6. *Fish and Seafood:* Aim to eat fish, particularly fatty fish like salmon, mackerel, and sardines, at least twice a week. They are high in omega-3 fatty acids, which are beneficial for heart health.

7. Poultry: Chicken and turkey are good protein sources and can be included in moderation. Choose skinless and opt for cooking methods like grilling, baking, or broiling.

8. Dairy: Low-fat or fat-free dairy products like yogurt, milk, and cheese provide calcium and protein. Choose unsalted or low-sodium options when available.

9. Herbs and Spices: Use a variety of herbs and spices to add flavor to dishes without the need for salt.

By incorporating these key components into your diet, you can enjoy the health benefits of the Mediterranean diet while also keeping your sodium intake in check.

The Importance of Fresh and Whole Foods

In the low sodium Mediterranean diet, the emphasis on fresh and whole foods is paramount. These foods are the cornerstone of the diet, providing essential nutrients, vitamins, minerals, and fiber, all of which contribute to overall health and well-being. Here's why fresh and whole foods are so important in this diet:

1. Nutrient Density: Fresh fruits, vegetables, whole grains, and legumes are packed with nutrients that are vital for maintaining health. They provide antioxidants, which protect against cell damage, as well as vitamins and minerals that support various bodily functions.

2. Low in Sodium: Naturally, fresh and whole foods contain little to no sodium. This makes them ideal for a low sodium diet, as they help keep overall sodium intake in check.

3. Fiber Content: Whole foods are rich in dietary fiber, which is beneficial for digestive health, helps control blood sugar levels, and can aid in weight management. Fiber also plays a role in reducing cholesterol levels and lowering the risk of heart disease.

4. Heart Health: The combination of healthy fats, fiber, and antioxidants found in fresh and whole foods supports heart health by reducing inflammation, lowering cholesterol levels, and improving blood vessel function.

5. Variety and Flavor: Incorporating a wide variety of fresh and whole foods into your diet ensures a diverse range of flavors and textures, making meals more enjoyable and satisfying.

To make the most of the low sodium Mediterranean diet, focus on incorporating fresh and whole foods into your meals as much as possible. Choose seasonal fruits and vegetables for peak flavor and nutrition, opt for whole grains instead of refined ones, and select lean proteins like fish and poultry.

Using Herbs and Spices for Flavor

One of the hallmarks of the low sodium Mediterranean diet is the use of herbs and spices to enhance the flavor of dishes without the need for added salt. This not only helps to keep sodium intake in check but also adds depth and complexity to your meals. Here are some tips for using herbs and spices in your cooking:

1. Experiment with Fresh Herbs: Fresh herbs like basil, cilantro, parsley, rosemary, thyme, and oregano can add a burst of flavor to any dish. Use them in salads, marinades, sauces, and as garnishes.

2. Explore Dried Spices: Dried spices like cumin, paprika, turmeric, coriander, and cinnamon can add warmth and richness to your cooking. They're perfect for seasoning meats, vegetables, and grains.

3. Make Your Own Blends: Create your own spice blends to have on hand for easy seasoning. For example, mix together dried oregano, thyme, basil, and garlic powder for a Mediterranean-inspired blend.

4. Use Citrus Zest and Juice: The zest and juice of lemons, limes, and oranges can add a fresh, tangy flavor to dishes without adding sodium. Use them in dressings, marinades, and to finish off cooked dishes.

5. Don't Forget Garlic and Onions: Garlic and onions are staples in Mediterranean cooking and can add depth of flavor to a variety of dishes. Use them as a base for soups, stews, and sauces.

6. Try Toasting Spices: Toasting spices in a dry pan before using them can intensify their flavor, making your dishes even more flavorful.

7. Balance Flavors: When using herbs and spices, aim for a balance of flavors. Start with small amounts and taste as you go, adjusting as needed to achieve the desired flavor profile.

By incorporating a variety of herbs and spices into your cooking, you can create delicious, low sodium dishes that are full of flavor and align with the principles of the Mediterranean diet. This approach not only enhances the taste of your meals but also provides additional health benefits, as many herbs and spices have antioxidant and anti-inflammatory properties.

4. SHOPPING AND PREPARATION TIPS

Adopting a low sodium Mediterranean diet requires some planning and preparation, both at the grocery store and in your kitchen. These tips will help you navigate the grocery store, read food labels for sodium content, and stock your pantry with low sodium Mediterranean essentials.

Navigating the Grocery Store

Shopping for a low sodium Mediterranean diet can be easy and enjoyable with a little bit of planning. Here are some tips for navigating the grocery store:

1. Make a List: Before heading to the store, plan your meals for the week and make a shopping list. This will help you stay focused and avoid impulse purchases that may not align with your diet.

2. Shop the Perimeter: Fresh produce, lean proteins, and dairy products are typically located around the perimeter of the store. Start your shopping here to fill your cart with fresh, whole foods.

3. *Choose Fresh or Frozen:* When it comes to fruits and vegetables, fresh or frozen options are usually lower in sodium than canned varieties. If you do choose canned, look for "no salt added" or "low sodium" labels.

4. Select Whole Grains: Opt for whole grain bread, pasta, and rice instead of refined options. Check the labels to ensure they are low in sodium.

5. *Pick Lean Proteins:* Choose fresh or frozen fish, poultry, and lean cuts of meat. Avoid processed meats like bacon, sausage, and deli meats, which are often high in sodium.

6. *Be Selective with Dairy:* Look for low-fat or fat-free dairy products, such as milk, yogurt, and cheese. Check the sodium content on the label and choose options with lower sodium levels.

7. *Read Labels on Packaged Foods:* Even seemingly healthy packaged foods can be high in sodium. Always check the nutrition labels and ingredient lists to make informed choices.

By following these tips, you can navigate the grocery store with confidence and fill your cart with low sodium Mediterranean diet-friendly foods.

Reading Food Labels for Sodium Content

Understanding how to read food labels is crucial for managing your sodium intake. Here's what to look for when checking labels for sodium content:

1. Serving Size: Always check the serving size first. The sodium content listed on the label is based on this amount, not necessarily the entire package.

2. Sodium Content: Look for the amount of sodium per serving, which is usually listed in milligrams (mg). Compare this to your daily sodium limit to determine if the food fits into your low sodium diet.

3. Percent Daily Value (%DV): The %DV tells you how much of the daily recommended intake of sodium a serving of the food provides. A %DV of 5% or less is considered low in sodium, while a %DV of 20% or more is considered high.

4. Low Sodium Claims: Foods labeled as "low sodium" contain 140 mg or less of sodium per serving. "Very low sodium" means 35 mg or less per serving, and "sodium-free" means less than 5 mg per serving.

5. *No Salt Added or Unsalted:* These labels indicate that no salt has been added during processing, but the food may still contain natural sodium. Check the nutrition facts to be sure.

6. *Ingredients List*: Sodium can appear under various names, such as salt, sodium chloride, monosodium glutamate (MSG), baking soda, and sodium nitrate. Scan the ingredients list for these terms to identify sources of sodium.

By becoming proficient at reading food labels, you can make informed choices that align with your low sodium Mediterranean diet goals.

Stocking Your Low Sodium Mediterranean Pantry

Having a well-stocked pantry is key to successfully following a low sodium Mediterranean diet. Here are some essentials to keep on hand:

*1. **Whole Grains:*** Stock up on whole grains like quinoa, brown rice, whole wheat pasta, and farro. These provide a good base for meals and are naturally low in sodium.

*2. **Legumes:*** Keep a variety of dried or low-sodium canned beans, lentils, and chickpeas. They're great for adding protein and fiber to salads, soups, and stews.

*3. **Nuts and Seeds:*** Almonds, walnuts, chia seeds, and flaxseeds are excellent sources of healthy fats and can be used to add crunch and flavor to dishes.

*4. **Herbs and Spices:*** Fill your spice rack with a variety of herbs and spices to flavor your meals without the need for salt. Consider growing your own herbs for the freshest flavors.

*5. **Olive Oil:*** Extra virgin olive oil is a staple in Mediterranean cooking. Use it for cooking, dressings, and drizzling over finished dishes.

*6. **Vinegars:*** Balsamic, red wine, and apple cider vinegars add acidity and brightness to salads and cooked dishes.

7. *Canned Tomatoes:* Look for no-salt-added or low-sodium canned tomatoes to use in sauces, soups, and stews.

8. *Whole Grain Breads and Crackers:* Choose whole grain options with low sodium content for sandwiches and snacks.

9. *Unsalted Broths:* Keep low-sodium vegetable, chicken, or beef broth on hand for soups and cooking grains.

10. *Fresh and Frozen Produce:* Stock your fridge and freezer with a variety of fruits and vegetables for easy access to nutrient-rich ingredients.

By keeping these low sodium Mediterranean essentials in your pantry, you'll be well-equipped to prepare healthy, flavorful meals that support your dietary goals.

5. RECIPES

BREAKFAST DELIGHTS

1. Mediterranean Morning Frittata

- *Prep time: 10 minutes*
- *Cook time: 20 minutes*
- *Serving size: 3 servings*

Ingredients:

- 8 large eggs
- 1/4 cup low-fat milk
- 1/2 cup diced bell peppers (red, yellow, or green)
- 1/4 cup diced red onion
- 1/2 cup chopped spinach
- 1/4 cup crumbled feta cheese
- 2 tablespoons chopped fresh basil
- 1 tablespoon olive oil
- 1/4 teaspoon black pepper

Nutritional facts (per serving):

- Calories: 215 kcal

- Protein: 14g

- Fat: 15g

- Carbohydrates: 6g

- Fiber: 1g

- Sodium: 220mg

Preparation directions:

1. Preheat the oven to 375°F (190°C).

2. In a medium bowl, whisk together the eggs and milk.

3. Stir in the bell peppers, red onion, spinach, feta cheese, basil, and black pepper.

4. Heat the olive oil in an oven-safe skillet over medium heat. Pour in the egg mixture and cook for 5 minutes, or until the edges begin to set.

5. Transfer the skillet to the oven and bake for 15 minutes, or until the frittata is set and lightly golden on top.

6. Remove from the oven, let cool for a few minutes, then slice and serve.

Variations/Substitutions:

- For a dairy-free version, omit the feta cheese or use a dairy-free cheese alternative.

- Add diced tomatoes or olives for extra Mediterranean flavor.

Health Benefit:

This Mediterranean Morning Frittata is a fantastic low sodium breakfast option that is rich in protein and vegetables. The inclusion of spinach provides a good source of vitamins A and C, while the eggs offer high-quality protein and healthy fats. The feta cheese adds a tangy flavor without significantly increasing the sodium content. This balanced meal supports heart health and provides sustained energy throughout the morning.

2. Greek Yogurt Parfait with Honey and Nuts

- Prep time: 5 minutes

- Serving size: 1 serving

Ingredients:

- 1 cup low-fat Greek yogurt

- 2 tablespoons honey

- 1/4 cup mixed nuts (almonds, walnuts, pistachios), chopped

- 1/2 cup mixed berries (strawberries, blueberries, raspberries)

Nutritional facts (per serving):

- Calories: 350 kcal

- Protein: 20g

- Fat: 15g

- Carbohydrates: 36g

- Fiber: 4g

- Sodium: 60mg

Preparation directions:

1. In a serving glass or bowl, layer half of the Greek yogurt.

2. Drizzle 1 tablespoon of honey over the yogurt.

3. Add a layer of mixed nuts and half of the berries.

4. Repeat the layers with the remaining yogurt, honey, nuts, and berries.

5. Serve immediately and enjoy.

Variations/Substitutions:

- Use agave syrup or maple syrup instead of honey for a different sweetness.

- Substitute the mixed nuts with granola for added crunch.

Health Benefit:

The Greek Yogurt Parfait with Honey and Nuts is a nutritious and delicious low sodium breakfast option. Greek yogurt is an excellent source of protein and calcium, while the nuts provide healthy fats and a satisfying crunch. Berries add natural sweetness and are packed with antioxidants, which can help protect against inflammation and disease. This parfait is a great way to start your day with a balanced combination of protein, healthy fats, and carbohydrates.

3. Olive and Tomato Breakfast Toast

- Prep time: 5 minutes

- Cook time: 2 minutes

- Serving size: 1 serving

Ingredients:

- 1 slice whole grain bread

- 2 tablespoons hummus

- 1/4 cup cherry tomatoes, halved

- 1 tablespoon sliced Kalamata olives

- 1 teaspoon chopped fresh parsley

- 1/4 teaspoon black pepper

Nutritional facts (per serving):

- Calories: 180 kcal

- Protein: 6g

- Fat: 6g

- Carbohydrates: 26g

- Fiber: 5g

- Sodium: 200mg

Preparation directions:

1. Toast the whole grain bread to your desired level of crispiness.
2. Spread the hummus evenly over the toasted bread.
3. Top with cherry tomatoes, Kalamata olives, and chopped parsley.
4. Sprinkle black pepper over the top and serve immediately.

Variations/Substitutions:

- Swap out hummus for avocado spread for a creamier texture.
- Add a drizzle of balsamic glaze for extra flavor.

Health Benefit:

The Olive and Tomato Breakfast Toast is a quick and easy low sodium option that provides a good balance of complex carbohydrates, protein, and healthy fats. Whole grain bread offers dietary fiber for digestive health, while hummus adds plant-based protein and heart-healthy fats. The addition of tomatoes and olives contributes antioxidants and vitamins, making this a nutritious and satisfying breakfast choice.

4. Spinach and Mushroom Omelette

- Prep time: 5 minutes

- Cook time: 10 minutes

- Serving size: 1 serving

Ingredients:

- 3 large eggs

- 1/4 cup chopped fresh spinach

- 1/4 cup sliced mushrooms

- 1 tablespoon diced red onion

- 1 tablespoon crumbled feta cheese

- 1 teaspoon olive oil

- 1/4 teaspoon black pepper

Nutritional facts (per serving):

- Calories: 230 kcal

- Protein: 18g

- Fat: 16g

- Carbohydrates: 4g

- Fiber: 1g

- Sodium: 220mg

Preparation directions:

1. In a bowl, whisk the eggs and black pepper together.
2. Heat the olive oil in a non-stick skillet over medium heat.
3. Sauté the mushrooms and red onion in the skillet for 2-3 minutes until softened.
4. Pour the whisked eggs over the sautéed vegetables.
5. Once the edges of the omelette start to set, sprinkle the chopped spinach and feta cheese over one half of the omelette.
6. Carefully fold the other half of the omelette over the filling.
7. Cook for an additional 2-3 minutes until the eggs are fully set and the cheese is slightly melted.
8. Slide the omelette onto a plate and serve.

Variations/Substitutions:

- Substitute the feta cheese with goat cheese for a different flavor.
- Add diced bell peppers for extra crunch and color.

Health Benefit:

The Spinach and Mushroom Omelette is a protein-packed low sodium breakfast that's also rich in vitamins and minerals. Eggs provide high-quality protein and essential nutrients, while spinach offers iron, folate, and vitamins A and C. Mushrooms contribute additional nutrients and antioxidants, making this omelette a healthy and satisfying start to your day.

5. Avocado and Egg Breakfast Bowl

- *Prep time: 10 minutes*
- *Cook time: 5 minutes*
- *Serving size: 1 serving*

Ingredients:
- 1/2 ripe avocado, sliced
- 1 large egg
- 1/2 cup cooked quinoa
- 1/4 cup cherry tomatoes, halved
- 1/4 cup baby spinach
- 1 tablespoon chopped red onion
- 1 tablespoon chopped fresh cilantro
- 1 teaspoon lemon juice
- 1/4 teaspoon black pepper
- 1/4 teaspoon paprika (optional)

***Nutritional facts (per serving):**

- Calories: 320 kcal

- Protein: 11g

- Fat: 19g

- Carbohydrates: 27g

- Fiber: 7g

- Sodium: 80mg

***Preparation directions:**

1. Cook the quinoa according to package instructions and set aside.

2. In a non-stick skillet, fry the egg to your desired doneness.

3. In a bowl, arrange the cooked quinoa, sliced avocado, cherry tomatoes, and baby spinach.

4. Top the bowl with the fried egg, chopped red onion, and fresh cilantro.

5. Drizzle lemon juice over the bowl and sprinkle with black pepper and paprika, if desired.

6. Gently mix the ingredients together before eating, or enjoy as is.

Variations/Substitutions:

- Substitute quinoa with brown rice or farro for a different whole grain option.
- Add a dollop of Greek yogurt for extra creaminess and protein.

Health Benefit:

The Avocado and Egg Breakfast Bowl is a nutrient-dense, low sodium meal that provides a balanced mix of healthy fats, protein, and fiber. Avocado is a great source of monounsaturated fats, which are beneficial for heart health. Eggs provide high-quality protein, while quinoa adds a complete protein source with all nine essential amino acids. This breakfast bowl is also packed with vitamins and minerals from the vegetables, making it an excellent choice for starting your day with energy and nourishment.

6. Lemon Ricotta Pancakes

- Prep time: 10 minutes

- Cook time: 10 minutes

- Serving size: 4 servings (2 pancakes per serving)

Ingredients:

- 1 cup whole wheat flour

- 1/2 cup low-fat ricotta cheese

- 3/4 cup low-fat milk

- 2 large eggs

- 2 tablespoons honey

- 1 tablespoon lemon zest

- 1 teaspoon baking powder

- 1/4 teaspoon baking soda

- 1/4 teaspoon salt

- Cooking spray or 1 teaspoon olive oil for the pan

Nutritional facts (per serving):

- Calories: 210 kcal

- Protein: 11g

- Fat: 5g

- Carbohydrates: 32g

- Fiber: 3g

- Sodium: 240mg

Preparation directions:

1. In a large mixing bowl, whisk together the whole wheat flour, baking powder, baking soda, and salt.
2. In another bowl, combine the ricotta cheese, milk, eggs, honey, and lemon zest.
3. Add the wet ingredients to the dry ingredients and stir until just combined.
4. Heat a non-stick skillet or griddle over medium heat and lightly coat with cooking spray or olive oil.
5. Pour 1/4 cup of batter onto the skillet for each pancake. Cook until bubbles form on the surface, then flip and cook until golden brown on the other side.
6. Serve the pancakes warm with a drizzle of honey or fresh berries.

Variations/Substitutions:

-   Substitute the whole wheat flour with almond flour for a gluten-free option.
-   Add a handful of blueberries to the batter for extra sweetness and antioxidants.

Health Benefit:

Lemon Ricotta Pancakes are a delightful and nutritious way to start your day. The whole wheat flour provides fiber for digestive health, while the ricotta cheese adds a creamy texture and a good source of protein. The lemon zest not only adds a refreshing flavor but also provides vitamin C, which supports the immune system. These pancakes are a great option for a low sodium Mediterranean breakfast that satisfies both taste and nutrition.

7. Mediterranean Breakfast Quinoa

- Prep time: 5 minutes

- Cook time: 15 minutes

- Serving size: 2 servings

Ingredients:

- 1/2 cup dry quinoa

- 1 cup water

- 1/4 cup chopped dried apricots

- 2 tablespoons chopped almonds

- 2 tablespoons pomegranate seeds

- 1 tablespoon honey

- 1/2 teaspoon ground cinnamon

- 1/4 teaspoon ground nutmeg

Nutritional facts (per serving):

- Calories: 280 kcal

- Protein: 8g

- Fat: 6g

- Carbohydrates: 50g

- Fiber: 6g

- Sodium: 10mg

Preparation directions:

1. Rinse the quinoa under cold water and drain.

2. In a medium saucepan, bring the quinoa and water to a boil. Reduce heat to low, cover, and simmer for 15 minutes, or until the quinoa is cooked and the water is absorbed.

3. Fluff the quinoa with a fork and stir in the chopped dried apricots, almonds, pomegranate seeds, honey, cinnamon, and nutmeg.

4. Serve warm, and enjoy a nutritious Mediterranean-inspired breakfast.

Variations/Substitutions:

- Substitute the dried apricots with dried figs or raisins for a different flavor.

- Use walnuts or pistachios instead of almonds for a variation in texture and taste.

Health Benefit:

Mediterranean Breakfast Quinoa is a wholesome and satisfying meal that provides a good balance of complex carbohydrates, protein, and healthy fats. Quinoa is a complete protein, offering all nine essential amino acids, making it an excellent choice for vegetarians and vegans. The addition of dried apricots, almonds, and pomegranate seeds adds natural sweetness, crunch, and a boost of antioxidants, supporting overall health and well-being.

8. Almond and Date Overnight Oats

- Prep time: 5 minutes (plus overnight soaking)
- Serving size: 1 serving

Ingredients:
- 1/2 cup rolled oats
- 3/4 cup unsweetened almond milk
- 4 pitted dates, chopped
- 2 tablespoons chopped almonds
- 1 tablespoon chia seeds
- 1/2 teaspoon vanilla extract
- 1/4 teaspoon ground cinnamon

Nutritional facts (per serving):

- Calories: 350 kcal

- Protein: 9g

- Fat: 11g

- Carbohydrates: 56g

- Fiber: 9g

- Sodium: 90mg

Preparation directions:

1. In a mason jar or airtight container, combine the rolled oats, almond milk, chopped dates, chopped almonds, chia seeds, vanilla extract, and ground cinnamon.

2. Stir well to ensure all the ingredients are evenly mixed.

3. Seal the container and refrigerate overnight or for at least 6 hours.

4. In the morning, give the oats a good stir, and add a splash of almond milk if needed to adjust the consistency.

5. Serve cold or at room temperature, and enjoy a hearty and nutritious breakfast.

Variations/Substitutions:

- Substitute almond milk with any other plant-based milk of your choice.
- Add a tablespoon of almond butter or peanut butter for extra creaminess and protein.

Health Benefit:

Almond and Date Overnight Oats are a convenient and healthy breakfast option, rich in fiber, protein, and healthy fats. The oats provide a slow-release of energy, keeping you full and satisfied throughout the morning. Dates offer natural sweetness and are a good source of potassium, while almonds and chia seeds add crunch and essential omega-3 fatty acids. This recipe is perfect for a low sodium Mediterranean diet, promoting heart health and overall well-being.

9. Shakshuka with Feta

- Prep time: 10 minutes

- Cook time: 20 minutes

- Serving size: 2 servings

Ingredients:

- 1 tablespoon olive oil

- 1/2 cup diced onion

- 1/2 cup diced bell pepper (any color)

- 2 cloves garlic, minced

- 1 cup canned no-salt-added diced tomatoes

- 1/2 teaspoon ground cumin

- 1/4 teaspoon paprika

- 1/4 teaspoon black pepper

- 4 large eggs

- 1/4 cup crumbled feta cheese

- 2 tablespoons chopped fresh parsley

Nutritional facts (per serving):

- Calories: 270 kcal

- Protein: 15g

- Fat: 18g

- Carbohydrates: 14g

- Fiber: 3g

- Sodium: 300mg

Preparation directions:

1. Heat the olive oil in a skillet over medium heat. Add the diced onion and bell pepper, and sauté for 5 minutes until softened.

2. Add the minced garlic, diced tomatoes, ground cumin, paprika, and black pepper. Stir well and simmer for 10 minutes until the sauce thickens.

3. Make four wells in the sauce and crack an egg into each well. Cover the skillet and cook for 5-7 minutes, or until the eggs are set to your desired consistency.

4. Sprinkle the crumbled feta cheese and chopped parsley over the top.

5. Serve the shakshuka hot, with whole grain bread or pita on the side for dipping.

Variations/Substitutions:

- Add a pinch of chili flakes for a spicy kick.
- Substitute feta cheese with goat cheese for a different flavor profile.

Health Benefit:

Shakshuka with Feta is a flavorful and nutritious dish that fits perfectly into a low sodium Mediterranean diet. The tomatoes provide a rich source of vitamins and antioxidants, while the eggs offer high-quality protein. Feta cheese adds a tangy taste without significantly increasing the sodium content. This dish is a great way to start your day with a balance of protein, healthy fats, and vegetables, supporting heart health and overall wellness.

10. Cucumber and Yogurt Smoothie

- *Prep time: 5 minutes*
- *Serving size: 1 serving*

Ingredients:

- 1/2 cup diced cucumber

- 1/2 cup low-fat Greek yogurt

- 1/4 cup unsweetened almond milk

- 1 tablespoon fresh mint leaves

- 1 teaspoon honey

- 1/2 teaspoon lemon juice

- Ice cubes (optional)

Nutritional facts (per serving):

- Calories: 100 kcal

- Protein: 8g

- Fat: 2g

- Carbohydrates: 12g

- Fiber: 1 g

- Sodium: 45mg

Preparation directions:

1. Place the diced cucumber, Greek yogurt, almond milk, fresh mint leaves, honey, and lemon juice into a blender.
2. Add a few ice cubes if desired for a chilled smoothie.
3. Blend until smooth and creamy.
4. Pour the smoothie into a glass and garnish with a sprig of mint or a slice of cucumber.

Variations/Substitutions:

- Add a scoop of protein powder for an extra protein boost.
- Substitute honey with agave syrup for a vegan option.

Health Benefit:

The Cucumber and Yogurt Smoothie is a refreshing and hydrating breakfast option, perfect for a low sodium Mediterranean diet. Cucumbers are high in water content and provide a cooling effect, while Greek yogurt adds a creamy texture and is a great source of probiotics and protein. The addition of mint and lemon enhances the flavor and aids in digestion. This smoothie is a light and healthy way to start your day, supporting digestive health and hydration.

11. Greek Salad with Lemon Dressing

- Prep time: 15 minutes

- Serving size: 4 servings

Ingredients:

- 4 cups chopped romaine lettuce

- 1 cup cherry tomatoes, halved

- 1 cup diced cucumber

- 1/2 cup sliced red onion

- 1/2 cup pitted Kalamata olives

- 1/2 cup crumbled feta cheese

- For the Lemon Dressing:

  - 1/4 cup extra virgin olive oil

  - 2 tablespoons fresh lemon juice

  - 1 teaspoon dried oregano

  - 1/2 teaspoon black pepper

Nutritional facts (per serving):

- Calories: 220 kcal

- Protein: 5g

- Fat: 19g

- Carbohydrates: 9g

- Fiber: 2g

- Sodium: 320mg

Preparation directions:

1. In a large bowl, combine the chopped romaine lettuce, cherry tomatoes, diced cucumber, sliced red onion, Kalamata olives, and crumbled feta cheese.

2. In a small bowl, whisk together the extra virgin olive oil, fresh lemon juice, dried oregano, and black pepper to make the dressing.

3. Drizzle the dressing over the salad and toss gently to coat all the ingredients.

4. Serve the Greek Salad immediately, garnished with additional feta cheese and olives if desired.

Variations/Substitutions:

- Add grilled chicken or chickpeas for extra protein.
- Substitute lemon juice with red wine vinegar for a different tangy flavor.

Health Benefit:

This Greek Salad with Lemon Dressing is a classic Mediterranean dish that's low in sodium and packed with fresh, nutrient-rich ingredients. The salad provides a good source of vitamins A and C from the vegetables, calcium from the feta cheese, and healthy fats from the olives and olive oil. The lemon dressing adds a refreshing and tangy flavor without the need for added salt, making it a heart-healthy choice for a low sodium diet.

12. Lentil and Vegetable Soup

- Prep time: 10 minutes

- Cook time: 30 minutes

- Serving size: 4 servings

Ingredients:

- 1 cup dried green lentils, rinsed

- 1 tablespoon olive oil

- 1 onion, diced

- 2 carrots, diced

- 2 celery stalks, diced

- 3 garlic cloves, minced

- 1 teaspoon ground cumin

- 1/2 teaspoon ground turmeric

- 1/2 teaspoon black pepper

- 4 cups low-sodium vegetable broth

- 1 can (14.5 oz) no-salt-added diced tomatoes

- 2 cups chopped kale or spinach

- 1 tablespoon lemon juice

__Nutritional facts (per serving):__

- Calories: 250 kcal

- Protein: 14g

- Fat: 5g

- Carbohydrates: 40g

- Fiber: 16g

- Sodium: 200mg

__Preparation directions:__

1. Heat the olive oil in a large pot over medium heat. Add the diced onion, carrots, and celery, and sauté for 5 minutes until the vegetables start to soften.

2. Add the minced garlic, ground cumin, ground turmeric, and black pepper, and cook for an additional minute, stirring constantly.

3. Stir in the rinsed lentils, low-sodium vegetable broth, and no-salt-added diced tomatoes. Bring the mixture to a boil, then reduce the heat to low and simmer for 20 minutes, or until the lentils are tender.

4. Add the chopped kale or spinach and cook for another 5 minutes until the greens are wilted.

5. Stir in the lemon juice and adjust the seasoning if needed.

6. Serve the Lentil and Vegetable Soup hot, with a slice of whole grain bread if desired.

Variations/Substitutions:

- Use different types of lentils, such as red or brown lentils, for variety.
- Add diced potatoes or sweet potatoes for a heartier soup.

Health Benefit:

Lentil and Vegetable Soup is a comforting and nutritious meal that's perfect for a low sodium Mediterranean diet. Lentils are an excellent source of plant-based protein and fiber, which can help lower cholesterol and improve heart health. The addition of vegetables and spices provides vitamins, minerals, and antioxidants, while the lemon juice adds a bright and tangy flavor. This soup is a great way to warm up and nourish your body with wholesome ingredients.

13. Quinoa Tabbouleh Salad

- Prep time: 15 minutes

- Cook time: 15 minutes

- Serving size: 4 servings

Ingredients:

- 1 cup quinoa, rinsed

- 2 cups water

- 1 cup chopped fresh parsley

- 1/2 cup chopped fresh mint

- 1 cup diced tomatoes

- 1 cup diced cucumber

- 1/4 cup diced red onion

- 1/4 cup lemon juice

- 2 tablespoons olive oil

- 1/4 teaspoon black pepper

Nutritional facts (per serving):

- Calories: 240 kcal

- Protein: 8g

- Fat: 8g

- Carbohydrates: 36g

- Fiber: 5g

- Sodium: 15mg

Preparation directions:

1. In a medium saucepan, bring the water to a boil. Add the rinsed quinoa, reduce the heat to low, cover, and simmer for 15 minutes, or until the quinoa is cooked and the water is absorbed.

2. Fluff the cooked quinoa with a fork and transfer it to a large bowl to cool.

3. Once the quinoa has cooled, add the chopped parsley, mint, tomatoes, cucumber, and red onion to the bowl.

4. In a small bowl, whisk together the lemon juice, olive oil, and black pepper to make the dressing.

5. Pour the dressing over the quinoa salad and toss gently to combine all the ingredients.

6. Serve the Quinoa Tabbouleh Salad chilled or at room temperature.

Variations/Substitutions:

- Add crumbled feta cheese or chickpeas for extra protein.

- Substitute lemon juice with lime juice for a different citrus flavor.

Health Benefit:

Quinoa Tabbouleh Salad is a fresh and light dish that's perfect for a low sodium Mediterranean diet. Quinoa is a complete protein source, providing all nine essential amino acids, making it an excellent choice for vegetarians and vegans. The salad is also packed with vitamins and antioxidants from the fresh herbs and vegetables, which can help reduce inflammation and promote heart health. The lemon and olive oil dressing adds a zesty flavor without the need for added salt.

14. Tomato and Cucumber Gazpacho

- Prep time: 15 minutes (plus chilling time)

- Serving size: 4 servings

Ingredients:

- 4 cups chopped ripe tomatoes

- 1 cup chopped cucumber

- 1/2 cup chopped red bell pepper

- 1/4 cup chopped red onion

- 2 cloves garlic, minced

- 2 tablespoons red wine vinegar

- 2 tablespoons olive oil

- 1/2 teaspoon black pepper

- 1 cup cold water

- Fresh basil leaves for garnish

Nutritional facts (per serving):

- Calories: 120 kcal

- Protein: 2g

- Fat: 7g

- Carbohydrates: 13g

- Fiber: 3g

- Sodium: 20mg

Preparation directions:

1. In a blender or food processor, combine the chopped tomatoes, cucumber, red bell pepper, red onion, garlic, red wine vinegar, olive oil, and black pepper.
2. Blend until the mixture is smooth, adding cold water as needed to reach the desired consistency.
3. Taste and adjust the seasoning if necessary.
4. Transfer the gazpacho to a container and refrigerate for at least 2 hours to allow the flavors to meld.
5. Serve the chilled gazpacho in bowls, garnished with fresh basil leaves.

Variations/Substitutions:

- Add a diced avocado to the soup before serving for creaminess and healthy fats.
- For a spicy kick, include a small jalapeño pepper in the blend.

Health Benefit:

Tomato and Cucumber Gazpacho is a refreshing and hydrating soup that's ideal for warm weather. Tomatoes are rich in lycopene, an antioxidant that has been linked to heart health and cancer prevention. Cucumbers add a cooling effect and are a good source of hydration, while the olive oil provides healthy monounsaturated fats. This gazpacho is a delicious way to enjoy a variety of vegetables in a low sodium, nutrient-dense meal.

15. White Bean and Arugula Salad

- Prep time: 10 minutes

- Serving size: 4 servings

Ingredients:

- 2 cups canned no-salt-added white beans, rinsed and drained

- 4 cups arugula

- 1 cup cherry tomatoes, halved

- 1/4 cup thinly sliced red onion

- 1/4 cup chopped fresh basil

- 2 tablespoons olive oil

- 2 tablespoons lemon juice

- 1/4 teaspoon black pepper

- 1/4 cup shaved Parmesan cheese (optional)

Nutritional facts (per serving):

- Calories: 180 kcal

- Protein: 8g

- Fat: 7g

- Carbohydrates: 23g

- Fiber: 6g

- Sodium: 30mg

Preparation directions:

1. In a large bowl, combine the white beans, arugula, cherry tomatoes, red onion, and fresh basil.
2. In a small bowl, whisk together the olive oil, lemon juice, and black pepper to make the dressing.
3. Pour the dressing over the salad and toss gently to coat all the ingredients.
4. Divide the salad among serving plates and top with shaved Parmesan cheese, if desired.
5. Serve immediately and enjoy a light and nutritious meal.

Variations/Substitutions:

- Substitute arugula with baby spinach or mixed greens for a different flavor profile.
- Add grilled chicken or tuna for added protein.

Health Benefit:

White Bean and Arugula Salad is a simple yet nutritious dish that aligns with the principles of the low sodium Mediterranean diet. White beans are an excellent source of plant-based protein and fiber, which can help improve digestive health and lower cholesterol levels. Arugula adds a peppery flavor and is rich in vitamins A, C, and K, supporting bone and immune health. The olive oil and lemon dressing provides healthy fats and a refreshing citrus taste, making this salad a heart-healthy choice.

16. Roasted Red Pepper and Almond Soup

- Prep time: 15 minutes

- Cook time: 25 minutes

- Serving size: 4 servings

Ingredients:

- 4 large red bell peppers, halved and seeded

- 1 tablespoon olive oil

- 1 onion, chopped

- 2 garlic cloves, minced

- 1/2 cup blanched almonds

- 4 cups low-sodium vegetable broth

- 1/2 teaspoon smoked paprika

- 1/4 teaspoon black pepper

- Fresh parsley for garnish

Nutritional facts (per serving):

- Calories: 180 kcal

- Protein: 5g

- Fat: 12g

- Carbohydrates: 15g

- Fiber: 4g

- Sodium: 100mg

Preparation directions:

1. Preheat the oven to 400°F (200°C). Place the red bell pepper halves on a baking sheet and roast for 20 minutes, or until the skins are charred and the peppers are tender.

2. Once cooled, peel the skins off the peppers and chop them into small pieces.

3. In a large pot, heat the olive oil over medium heat. Add the chopped onion and garlic, and sauté for 5 minutes until softened.

4. Add the roasted red peppers, blanched almonds, low-sodium vegetable broth, smoked paprika, and black pepper to the pot.

5. Bring the mixture to a boil, then reduce the heat and simmer for 15 minutes.

6. Use an immersion blender or transfer the soup to a blender and blend until smooth.

7. Serve the soup hot, garnished with fresh parsley.

Variations/Substitutions:

- Substitute almonds with cashews for a creamier texture.

- Add a dollop of Greek yogurt for a tangy flavor.

Health Benefit:

Roasted Red Pepper and Almond Soup is a flavorful and comforting dish that's perfect for a low sodium Mediterranean diet. Red bell peppers are high in vitamins A and C, which are powerful antioxidants that support immune function and skin health. Almonds add a nutty flavor and provide healthy fats, protein, and fiber. This soup is a great way to enjoy a warm and satisfying meal that's both nutritious and low in sodium.

17. Mediterranean Chickpea Salad

- Prep time: 15 minutes

- Serving size: 4 servings

Ingredients:

- 2 cups canned no-salt-added chickpeas, rinsed and drained

- 1 cup diced cucumber

- 1 cup halved cherry tomatoes

- 1/2 cup diced red bell pepper

- 1/4 cup thinly sliced red onion

- 1/4 cup chopped fresh parsley

- 1/4 cup crumbled feta cheese

- 2 tablespoons olive oil

- 2 tablespoons lemon juice

- 1/2 teaspoon dried oregano

- 1/4 teaspoon black pepper

Nutritional facts (per serving):

- Calories: 210 kcal

- Protein: 8g

- Fat: 10g

- Carbohydrates: 24g

- Fiber: 6g

- Sodium: 150mg

Preparation directions:

1. In a large bowl, combine the chickpeas, cucumber, cherry tomatoes, red bell pepper, red onion, and fresh parsley.

2. In a small bowl, whisk together the olive oil, lemon juice, dried oregano, and black pepper to make the dressing.

3. Pour the dressing over the salad and toss gently to coat all the ingredients.

4. Sprinkle the crumbled feta cheese over the top of the salad.

5. Serve the Mediterranean Chickpea Salad chilled or at room temperature.

Variations/Substitutions:

- Add sliced Kalamata olives for a briny flavor.

- Substitute feta cheese with goat cheese for a creamier texture.

Health Benefit:

Mediterranean Chickpea Salad is a vibrant and nutritious dish that's perfect for a low sodium Mediterranean diet. Chickpeas are an excellent source of plant-based protein and fiber, which can help regulate blood sugar levels and promote digestive health. The vegetables in the salad provide vitamins, minerals, and antioxidants, while the olive oil and feta cheese add healthy fats and calcium. This salad is a delicious way to enjoy a variety of nutrient-dense ingredients in a low sodium meal.

18. Eggplant and Tomato Salad

- *Prep time: 10 minutes*
- *Cook time: 20 minutes*
- *Serving size: 4 servings*

Ingredients:

- 1 large eggplant, sliced into 1/2-inch rounds

- 2 tablespoons olive oil

- 2 cups cherry tomatoes, halved

- 1/4 cup chopped fresh basil

- 2 tablespoons balsamic vinegar

- 1/4 teaspoon black pepper

- 1/4 cup crumbled feta cheese (optional)

Nutritional facts (per serving):

- Calories: 130 kcal

- Protein: 2g

- Fat: 8g

- Carbohydrates: 14g

- Fiber: 5g

- Sodium: 80mg

Preparation directions:

1. Preheat the oven to 400°F (200°C). Brush the eggplant slices with olive oil and place them on a baking sheet.

2. Roast the eggplant in the oven for 20 minutes, flipping halfway through, until tender and golden brown.

3. In a large bowl, combine the roasted eggplant, cherry tomatoes, and chopped fresh basil.

4. Drizzle the balsamic vinegar over the salad and toss gently to combine.

5. Season with black pepper and sprinkle crumbled feta cheese on top, if desired.

6. Serve the Eggplant and Tomato Salad warm or at room temperature.

Variations/Substitutions:

- Add sliced red onions or olives for extra flavor.
- Substitute balsamic vinegar with lemon juice for a citrusy dressing.

Health Benefit:

Eggplant and Tomato Salad is a light and flavorful dish that's ideal for a low sodium Mediterranean diet. Eggplant is a good source of fiber, vitamins, and antioxidants, which can help protect against chronic diseases. Tomatoes are rich in lycopene, an antioxidant that has been linked to heart health and cancer prevention. The addition of olive oil and balsamic vinegar provides healthy fats and a tangy flavor, making this salad a nutritious and delicious choice.

19. Carrot and Orange Soup

- Prep time: 10 minutes

- Cook time: 25 minutes

- Serving size: 4 servings

Ingredients:

- 1 tablespoon olive oil

- 1 onion, chopped

- 4 cups chopped carrots

- 4 cups low-sodium vegetable broth

- 1 cup orange juice

- 1 teaspoon ground ginger

- 1/4 teaspoon black pepper

- Fresh parsley for garnish

Nutritional facts (per serving):

- Calories: 130 kcal

- Protein: 2g

- Fat: 4g

- Carbohydrates: 22g

- Fiber: 5g

- Sodium: 150mg

Preparation directions:

1. Heat the olive oil in a large pot over medium heat. Add the chopped onion and sauté for 5 minutes until softened.

2. Add the chopped carrots to the pot and cook for another 5 minutes, stirring occasionally.

3. Pour in the low-sodium vegetable broth and orange juice. Bring the mixture to a boil, then reduce the heat and simmer for 15 minutes, or until the carrots are tender.

4. Use an immersion blender or transfer the soup to a blender and blend until smooth.

5. Stir in the ground ginger and black pepper, and adjust the seasoning if needed.

6. Serve the Carrot and Orange Soup hot, garnished with fresh parsley.

Variations/Substitutions:

-   Add a pinch of ground cinnamon or nutmeg for a warm spice flavor.

-   Substitute orange juice with apple juice for a different fruity twist.

Health Benefit:

Carrot and Orange Soup is a vibrant and nutritious dish that's perfect for a low sodium Mediterranean diet. Carrots are a great source of beta-carotene, which is converted into vitamin A in the body, supporting eye health and immune function. Orange juice adds a natural sweetness and provides vitamin C, an antioxidant that helps protect cells from damage. This soup is a delicious way to enjoy a variety of vitamins and minerals in a low sodium meal.

20. Beet and Goat Cheese Salad

- Prep time: 15 minutes

- Cook time: 45 minutes (for roasting beets)

- Serving size: 4 servings

Ingredients:

- 4 medium beets, roasted and sliced

- 4 cups mixed greens (such as arugula and spinach)

- 1/4 cup crumbled goat cheese

- 1/4 cup chopped walnuts

- 2 tablespoons balsamic vinegar

- 1 tablespoon olive oil

- 1/4 teaspoon black pepper

Nutritional facts (per serving):

- Calories: 200 kcal

- Protein: 6g

- Fat: 13g

- Carbohydrates: 16g

- Fiber: 4g

- Sodium: 125mg

Preparation directions:

1. Preheat the oven to 400°F (200°C). Wrap the whole beets in foil and roast in the oven for 45 minutes, or until tender. Let them cool, then peel and slice.

2. In a large bowl, arrange the mixed greens and top with the sliced roasted beets.

3. Sprinkle the crumbled goat cheese and chopped walnuts over the salad.

4. In a small bowl, whisk together the balsamic vinegar, olive oil, and black pepper to make the dressing.

5. Drizzle the dressing over the salad and toss gently to combine.

6. Serve the Beet and Goat Cheese Salad immediately, enjoying the combination of flavors and textures.

Variations/Substitutions:

- Substitute walnuts with pecans or almonds for a different crunch.

- Add sliced oranges or strawberries for a sweet and tangy contrast.

Health Benefit:

Beet and Goat Cheese Salad is a colorful and nutrient-rich dish that's ideal for a low sodium Mediterranean diet. Beets are high in fiber, vitamins, and minerals, and have been shown to support heart health and reduce inflammation. Goat cheese adds a creamy texture and a good source of protein, while walnuts provide healthy fats and antioxidants. This salad is a delightful way to enjoy a variety of nutrient-dense ingredients in a low sodium meal.

MAIN COURSES

21. Grilled Salmon with Lemon and Herbs

- *Prep time: 10 minutes*
- *Cook time: 10 minutes*
- *Serving size: 4 servings*

Ingredients:

- 4 salmon fillets (6 ounces each)
- 2 tablespoons olive oil
- 2 tablespoons fresh lemon juice
- 1 tablespoon chopped fresh dill
- 1 tablespoon chopped fresh parsley
- 1 garlic clove, minced
- 1/4 teaspoon black pepper
- Lemon slices for garnish

Nutritional facts (per serving):

- Calories: 280 kcal

- Protein: 34g

- Fat: 15g

- Carbohydrates: 1g

- Fiber: 0g

- Sodium: 75mg

Preparation directions:

1. Preheat the grill to medium-high heat.

2. In a small bowl, whisk together the olive oil, lemon juice, dill, parsley, garlic, and black pepper.

3. Brush the salmon fillets with the herb mixture on both sides.

4. Place the salmon on the grill, skin-side down, and cook for 5 minutes.

5. Flip the salmon and grill for another 5 minutes, or until the fish flakes easily with a fork.

6. Serve the grilled salmon with lemon slices and additional fresh herbs if desired.

Variations/Substitutions:

- Substitute dill and parsley with other fresh herbs like thyme or basil.

- Add a sprinkle of paprika or cayenne pepper for a bit of heat.

Health Benefit:

Grilled Salmon with Lemon and Herbs is a heart-healthy main course that's perfect for a low sodium Mediterranean diet. Salmon is rich in omega-3 fatty acids, which are beneficial for heart health and can help reduce inflammation. The fresh herbs and lemon add flavor without the need for added salt, making this dish a nutritious and delicious option for those looking to maintain a low sodium intake.

22. Vegetable Paella

- *Prep time: 15 minutes*
- *Cook time: 30 minutes*
- *Serving size: 4 servings*

Ingredients:

- 1 tablespoon olive oil

- 1 onion, chopped

- 2 garlic cloves, minced

- 1 red bell pepper, chopped

- 1 yellow bell pepper, chopped

- 1 cup Arborio rice

- 2 cups low-sodium vegetable broth

- 1 cup diced tomatoes

- 1 teaspoon smoked paprika

- 1/2 teaspoon saffron threads

- 1 cup frozen peas, thawed

- 1/4 cup chopped fresh parsley

- Lemon wedges for serving

Nutritional facts (per serving):

- Calories: 280 kcal

- Protein: 7g

- Fat: 5g

- Carbohydrates: 51g

- Fiber: 5g

- Sodium: 150mg

Preparation directions:

1. Heat the olive oil in a large skillet or paella pan over medium heat. Add the onion and garlic, and sauté for 5 minutes until softened.

2. Add the red and yellow bell peppers and cook for another 5 minutes.

3. Stir in the Arborio rice, coating it well with the oil and vegetables.

4. Pour in the low-sodium vegetable broth, diced tomatoes, smoked paprika, and saffron threads. Bring the mixture to a boil, then reduce the heat to low and simmer for 20

minutes, or until the rice is cooked and the liquid is absorbed.

5. Stir in the thawed peas and cook for an additional 5 minutes.

6. Remove from heat and let the paella rest for a few minutes. Sprinkle with chopped fresh parsley and serve with lemon wedges.

Variations/Substitutions:

- Add artichoke hearts or roasted red peppers for additional Mediterranean flavors.

- Substitute Arborio rice with brown rice for a whole grain option (note: cooking time may vary).

Health Benefit:

Vegetable Paella is a colorful and nutritious dish that's full of flavor without being high in sodium. The variety of vegetables provides an array of vitamins and antioxidants, while the Arborio rice offers a satisfying texture and energy. Saffron and smoked paprika add depth to the dish, making it a delightful low sodium option for a Mediterranean-inspired meal.

23. Baked Chicken with Olives and Tomatoes

- Prep time: 10 minutes

- Cook time: 25 minutes

- Serving size: 4 servings

Ingredients:

- 4 boneless, skinless chicken breasts

- 2 tablespoons olive oil

- 1 cup cherry tomatoes, halved

- 1/2 cup pitted Kalamata olives, halved

- 2 garlic cloves, minced

- 1 teaspoon dried oregano

- 1/4 teaspoon black pepper

- Fresh basil leaves for garnish

Nutritional facts (per serving):

- Calories: 240 kcal

- Protein: 26g

- Fat: 13g

- Carbohydrates: 4g

- Fiber: 1g

- Sodium: 200mg

Preparation directions:

1. Preheat the oven to 375°F (190°C).
2. Place the chicken breasts in a baking dish and drizzle with olive oil.
3. Scatter the cherry tomatoes, Kalamata olives, and minced garlic around the chicken.
4. Sprinkle the dried oregano and black pepper over the top.
5. Bake in the preheated oven for 25 minutes, or until the chicken is cooked through and the tomatoes are soft.
6. Garnish with fresh basil leaves before serving.

Variations/Substitutions:

- Add sliced bell peppers or onions for extra vegetables.
- Substitute dried oregano with fresh oregano or thyme for a different herb flavor.

Health Benefit:

Baked Chicken with Olives and Tomatoes is a Mediterranean-inspired dish that's low in sodium and high in flavor. The chicken provides a lean source of protein, while the olives and tomatoes add heart-healthy fats and antioxidants. This dish is a great way to enjoy a satisfying and nutritious meal that aligns with the principles of the low sodium Mediterranean diet.

24. Stuffed Bell Peppers with Quinoa

- *Prep time: 15 minutes*

- *Cook time: 30 minutes*

- *Serving size: 4 servings*

Ingredients:

- 4 large bell peppers, halved and seeded

- 1 cup cooked quinoa

- 1 cup canned no-salt-added black beans, rinsed and drained

- 1 cup corn kernels (fresh or frozen)

- 1/2 cup diced tomatoes

- 1/4 cup chopped fresh cilantro

- 2 tablespoons lime juice

- 1 teaspoon ground cumin

- 1/4 teaspoon black pepper

- 1/4 cup shredded low-fat cheddar cheese (optional)

Nutritional facts (per serving):

- Calories: 220 kcal

- Protein: 10g

- Fat: 3g

- Carbohydrates: 40g

- Fiber: 8g

- Sodium: 80mg

Preparation directions:

1. Preheat the oven to 375°F (190°C).
2. In a large bowl, mix together the cooked quinoa, black beans, corn kernels, diced tomatoes, chopped cilantro, lime juice, ground cumin, and black pepper.
3. Stuff each bell pepper half with the quinoa mixture, packing it tightly.
4. Place the stuffed bell peppers in a baking dish and cover with foil.
5. Bake in the preheated oven for 25 minutes. Remove the foil and sprinkle shredded cheddar cheese on top of each pepper, if desired.
6. Bake for an additional 5 minutes, or until the cheese is melted and the peppers are tender.
7. Serve the Stuffed Bell Peppers with Quinoa hot, garnished with extra cilantro if desired.

Variations/Substitutions:

-   Add diced avocado or a dollop of Greek yogurt on top for creaminess.
-   Substitute black beans with kidney beans or chickpeas for a different protein source.

Health Benefit:

Stuffed Bell Peppers with Quinoa are a colorful and nutritious main course that's perfect for a low sodium Mediterranean diet. Quinoa is a complete protein, providing all nine essential amino acids, and is also a good source of fiber. The black beans and corn add additional protein and fiber, while the bell peppers are rich in vitamins A and C. This dish is a great way to enjoy a variety of nutrient-dense ingredients in a low sodium, flavorful meal.

25. Eggplant Moussaka

- Prep time: 20 minutes

- Cook time: 45 minutes

- Serving size: 6 servings

Ingredients:

- 2 large eggplants, sliced into 1/4-inch rounds

- 2 tablespoons olive oil

- 1 onion, chopped

- 2 garlic cloves, minced

- 1 pound ground turkey or lean ground beef

- 1 can (14.5 oz) no-salt-added diced tomatoes

- 1 teaspoon dried oregano

- 1/2 teaspoon ground cinnamon

- 1/4 teaspoon black pepper

For the Béchamel Sauce:

  - 2 tablespoons unsalted butter

  - 2 tablespoons all-purpose flour

  - 1 1/2 cups low-fat milk

  - 1/4 teaspoon ground nutmeg

  - 1/2 cup grated Parmesan cheese

Nutritional facts (per serving):

- Calories: 300 kcal

- Protein: 22g

- Fat: 16g

- Carbohydrates: 20g

- Fiber: 6g

- Sodium: 150mg

Preparation directions:

1. Preheat the oven to 375°F (190°C).

2. Brush the eggplant slices with olive oil and place them on a baking sheet. Bake for 20 minutes, or until tender.

3. In a skillet, heat 1 tablespoon of olive oil over medium heat. Add the onion and garlic, and sauté for 5 minutes until softened.

4. Add the ground turkey or beef, and cook until browned. Stir in the diced tomatoes, oregano, cinnamon, and black pepper. Simmer for 10 minutes.

5. For the béchamel sauce, melt the butter in a saucepan over medium heat. Whisk in the flour and cook for 1 minute. Gradually add the milk, whisking constantly, until the sauce thickens. Stir in the nutmeg and Parmesan cheese.

6. In a baking dish, layer half of the eggplant slices, then spread half of the meat mixture on top. Repeat with the remaining eggplant and meat. Pour the béchamel sauce over the top.

7. Bake in the preheated oven for 25 minutes, or until the top is golden and bubbly.

8. Let the moussaka rest for 10 minutes before serving.

Variations/Substitutions:

- Use zucchini slices instead of eggplant for a different flavor.

- Substitute the ground turkey with lentils for a vegetarian option.

Health Benefit:

Eggplant Moussaka is a hearty and comforting dish that fits well into a low sodium Mediterranean diet. Eggplant is a good source of fiber, vitamins, and antioxidants. The ground turkey provides lean protein, while the béchamel sauce adds creaminess without excessive sodium. This dish is a great way to enjoy a traditional Mediterranean meal with a focus on heart-healthy ingredients.

26. Mediterranean Vegetable Stew

- *Prep time: 15 minutes*
- *Cook time: 30 minutes*
- *Serving size: 4 servings*

Ingredients:

- 1 tablespoon olive oil
- 1 onion, chopped
- 2 garlic cloves, minced
- 1 bell pepper, chopped
- 1 zucchini, chopped
- 1 eggplant, chopped
- 1 can (14.5 oz) no-salt-added diced tomatoes
- 1 cup low-sodium vegetable broth
- 1 teaspoon dried basil
- 1/2 teaspoon dried thyme
- 1/4 teaspoon black pepper
- 1/4 cup chopped fresh parsley

Nutritional facts (per serving):

- Calories: 120 kcal

- Protein: 3g

- Fat: 5g

- Carbohydrates: 18g

- Fiber: 6g

- Sodium: 80mg

Preparation directions:

1. Heat the olive oil in a large pot over medium heat. Add the onion and garlic, and sauté for 5 minutes until softened.

2. Add the bell pepper, zucchini, and eggplant to the pot. Cook for 10 minutes, stirring occasionally.

3. Stir in the diced tomatoes, vegetable broth, basil, thyme, and black pepper. Bring the mixture to a boil, then reduce the heat and simmer for 15 minutes, or until the vegetables are tender.

4. Remove from heat and stir in the fresh parsley.

5. Serve the Mediterranean Vegetable Stew hot, with a side of whole grain bread or over cooked quinoa.

Variations/Substitutions:

- Add chickpeas or white beans for added protein and texture.

- Substitute zucchini with yellow squash for a different flavor.

Health Benefit:

Mediterranean Vegetable Stew is a light and nutritious dish that's perfect for a low sodium Mediterranean diet. The variety of vegetables provides a wealth of vitamins, minerals, and fiber, which are essential for maintaining good health. The olive oil adds healthy fats, while the herbs and spices bring Mediterranean flavors to the dish without the need for added salt. This stew is a great way to enjoy a comforting and heart-healthy meal.

27. Lemon and Herb Baked Cod

- *Prep time: 10 minutes*

- *Cook time: 15 minutes*

- *Serving size: 4 servings*

Ingredients:

- 4 cod fillets (6 ounces each)

- 2 tablespoons olive oil

- 2 tablespoons fresh lemon juice

- 1 tablespoon chopped fresh parsley

- 1 tablespoon chopped fresh dill

- 2 garlic cloves, minced

- 1/4 teaspoon black pepper

- Lemon slices for garnish

Nutritional facts (per serving):

- Calories: 180 kcal

- Protein: 23g

- Fat: 9g

- Carbohydrates: 1g

- Fiber: 0g

- Sodium: 70mg

Preparation directions:

1. Preheat the oven to 400°F (200°C).
2. Place the cod fillets in a baking dish.
3. In a small bowl, whisk together the olive oil, lemon juice, parsley, dill, garlic, and black pepper.
4. Pour the herb mixture over the cod fillets, making sure they are well coated.
5. Bake in the preheated oven for 15 minutes, or until the fish flakes easily with a fork.
6. Serve the Lemon and Herb Baked Cod hot, garnished with lemon slices.

Variations/Substitutions:

- Substitute cod with another white fish like haddock or tilapia.

- Add a sprinkle of paprika or cayenne pepper for a bit of heat.

Health Benefit:

Lemon and Herb Baked Cod is a light and flavorful main course that's perfect for a low sodium Mediterranean diet. Cod is a lean source of protein and is rich in omega-3 fatty acids, which are beneficial for heart health. The combination of fresh herbs and lemon adds a burst of flavor without the need for added salt, making this dish a heart-healthy choice for those looking to maintain a low sodium intake.

28. Spinach and Feta Stuffed Chicken

- Prep time: 15 minutes

- Cook time: 25 minutes

- Serving size: 4 servings

Ingredients:

- 4 boneless, skinless chicken breasts

- 2 cups fresh spinach, chopped

- 1/2 cup crumbled feta cheese

- 2 tablespoons chopped sun-dried tomatoes

- 1 tablespoon olive oil

- 1/2 teaspoon black pepper

- Toothpicks or kitchen twine for securing

Nutritional facts (per serving):

- Calories: 240 kcal

- Protein: 29g

- Fat: 12g

- Carbohydrates: 3g

- Fiber: 1g

- Sodium: 320mg

Preparation directions:

1. Preheat the oven to 375°F (190°C).

2. Cut a pocket into each chicken breast, being careful not to cut all the way through.

3. In a bowl, mix together the chopped spinach, crumbled feta cheese, and sun-dried tomatoes.

4. Stuff each chicken breast with the spinach and feta mixture, then secure with toothpicks or kitchen twine.

5. Season the outside of the chicken breasts with black pepper.

6. Heat the olive oil in a skillet over medium heat. Sear the chicken breasts for 2-3 minutes on each side until golden brown.

7. Transfer the chicken to a baking dish and bake in the preheated oven for 20 minutes, or until the chicken is cooked through.

8. Serve the Spinach and Feta Stuffed Chicken hot, removing the toothpicks or twine before serving.

Variations/Substitutions:

- Add chopped olives or capers to the stuffing for a briny flavor.

- Substitute feta cheese with goat cheese for a creamier texture.

Health Benefit:

Spinach and Feta Stuffed Chicken is a delicious and nutritious main course that fits well into a low sodium Mediterranean diet. The chicken provides a lean source of protein, while the spinach is rich in iron and vitamins A and C. Feta cheese adds calcium and a tangy flavor without significantly increasing the sodium content. This dish is a great way to enjoy a flavorful and balanced meal that supports heart health.

29. Ratatouille with Herbed Couscous

- *Prep time: 20 minutes*
- *Cook time: 40 minutes*
- *Serving size: 4 servings*

Ingredients:

- 1 eggplant, diced

- 2 zucchinis, diced

- 1 bell pepper, diced

- 1 onion, chopped

- 2 garlic cloves, minced

- 1 can (14.5 oz) no-salt-added diced tomatoes

- 2 tablespoons olive oil

- 1 teaspoon dried thyme

- 1/2 teaspoon dried rosemary

- 1/4 teaspoon black pepper

- 1 cup whole wheat couscous

- 1 1/4 cups low-sodium vegetable broth

- 2 tablespoons chopped fresh parsley

Nutritional facts (per serving):
- Calories: 320 kcal

- Protein: 9g

- Fat: 9g

- Carbohydrates: 54g

- Fiber: 10g

- Sodium: 150mg

Preparation directions:
1. Preheat the oven to 375°F (190°C).

2. In a large bowl, combine the diced eggplant, zucchinis, bell pepper, onion, and minced garlic.

3. Drizzle the olive oil over the vegetables and toss to coat. Sprinkle with thyme, rosemary, and black pepper.

4. Spread the vegetables in a single layer on a baking sheet and roast in the oven for 30 minutes, stirring halfway through.

5. While the vegetables are roasting, prepare the couscous. Bring the low-sodium vegetable broth to a boil in a saucepan. Stir in the couscous, cover, and remove from heat. Let it stand for 5 minutes, then fluff with a fork.

6. Serve the roasted ratatouille over the herbed couscous and garnish with fresh parsley.

Variations/Substitutions:

- Add chickpeas or white beans to the ratatouille for added protein.
- Substitute couscous with quinoa or brown rice for a gluten-free option.

Health Benefit:

Ratatouille with Herbed Couscous is a vibrant and nutritious dish that's perfect for a low sodium Mediterranean diet. The variety of vegetables in the ratatouille provides a wealth of vitamins, minerals, and antioxidants, while the whole wheat couscous offers a good source of fiber and complex carbohydrates. This dish is a delicious way to enjoy a variety of nutrient-dense ingredients in a low sodium, flavorful meal that supports overall health and well-being.

30. Grilled Vegetable and Halloumi Skewers

- Prep time: 15 minutes

- Cook time: 10 minutes

- Serving size: 4 servings

Ingredients:

- 2 bell peppers (any color), cut into chunks

- 2 zucchinis, sliced into rounds

- 1 red onion, cut into chunks

- 8 ounces halloumi cheese, cut into cubes

- 2 tablespoons olive oil

- 1 tablespoon lemon juice

- 1 teaspoon dried oregano

- 1/4 teaspoon black pepper

- Wooden or metal skewers

Nutritional facts (per serving):

- Calories: 280 kcal

- Protein: 14g

- Fat: 20g

- Carbohydrates: 14g

- Fiber: 3g

- Sodium: 400mg

Preparation directions:

1. Preheat the grill to medium-high heat.
2. Thread the bell pepper chunks, zucchini rounds, red onion chunks, and halloumi cubes onto skewers, alternating between vegetables and cheese.
3. In a small bowl, whisk together the olive oil, lemon juice, oregano, and black pepper.
4. Brush the skewers with the olive oil mixture.
5. Grill the skewers for 5 minutes on each side, or until the vegetables are tender and the halloumi is golden brown.
6. Serve the Grilled Vegetable and Halloumi Skewers hot, with extra lemon wedges on the side.

Variations/Substitutions:

- Add cherry tomatoes or mushrooms to the skewers for added variety.
- Substitute halloumi with tofu for a vegan option.

Health Benefit:

Grilled Vegetable and Halloumi Skewers are a delightful and healthy option for a low sodium Mediterranean diet. The grilled vegetables provide essential vitamins and fiber, while the halloumi cheese adds a satisfying texture and a good source of protein. This dish is a great way to enjoy a variety of flavors and nutrients in a low sodium, heart-healthy meal that's perfect for outdoor grilling.

SIDES AND SNACKS

31. Hummus with Roasted Vegetables

- *Prep time: 15 minutes*
- *Cook time: 25 minutes*
- *Serving size: 4 servings*

Ingredients:

- 1 cup homemade or store-bought low-sodium hummus
- 2 bell peppers (any color), sliced
- 2 zucchinis, sliced
- 1 eggplant, sliced
- 2 tablespoons olive oil
- 1/4 teaspoon black pepper
- Fresh parsley for garnish

Nutritional facts (per serving):

- Calories: 220 kcal
- Protein: 8g
- Fat: 14g

- Carbohydrates: 20g

- Fiber: 8g

- Sodium: 150mg

Preparation directions:

1. Preheat the oven to 400°F (200°C).
2. Place the sliced bell peppers, zucchinis, and eggplant on a baking sheet. Drizzle with olive oil and sprinkle with black pepper.
3. Roast the vegetables in the oven for 25 minutes, or until tender and slightly charred.
4. Arrange the roasted vegetables on a platter and serve with a bowl of hummus for dipping.
5. Garnish with fresh parsley before serving.

Variations/Substitutions:

-   Add other vegetables like cherry tomatoes or asparagus for variety.
-   Use flavored hummus, such as roasted red pepper or garlic, for added taste.

Health Benefit:

Hummus with Roasted Vegetables is a delicious and nutritious snack that's perfect for a low sodium Mediterranean diet. Hummus provides a good source of plant-based protein and fiber, while the roasted vegetables offer vitamins, minerals, and antioxidants. This dish is a great way to enjoy a variety of nutrient-dense ingredients in a low sodium, flavorful snack.

32. Tzatziki with Cucumber Slices

- *Prep time: 10 minutes*
- *Chill time: 1 hour*
- *Serving size: 4 servings*

Ingredients:

- 1 cup low-fat Greek yogurt
- 1 cucumber, grated and squeezed dry
- 2 garlic cloves, minced
- 1 tablespoon fresh dill, chopped
- 1 tablespoon lemon juice
- 1/4 teaspoon black pepper
- Cucumber slices for serving

Nutritional facts (per serving):

- Calories: 60 kcal
- Protein: 6g
- Fat: 1g

- Carbohydrates: 7g

- Fiber: 1g

- Sodium: 40mg

Preparation directions:

1. In a bowl, combine the Greek yogurt, grated cucumber, minced garlic, chopped dill, lemon juice, and black pepper.
2. Mix well until all the ingredients are evenly distributed.
3. Cover the bowl and refrigerate the tzatziki for at least 1 hour to allow the flavors to meld.
4. Serve the chilled tzatziki with cucumber slices for dipping.

Variations/Substitutions:

- Add a pinch of ground cumin or mint for a different flavor.
- Serve with carrot sticks or bell pepper strips for added variety.

Health Benefit:

Tzatziki with Cucumber Slices is a light and refreshing snack that's ideal for a low sodium Mediterranean diet. Greek yogurt provides a creamy texture and is a good source of protein and probiotics, supporting digestive health. Cucumbers are hydrating and low in calories, making this snack a healthy choice for those looking to maintain a low sodium intake while enjoying a flavorful and nutritious treat.

33. Olive Tapenade on Whole Grain Crackers

- Prep time: 10 minutes

- Serving size: 4 servings

Ingredients:

- 1 cup pitted Kalamata olives

- 2 tablespoons capers, rinsed

- 1 garlic clove

- 2 tablespoons chopped fresh parsley

- 2 tablespoons olive oil

- 1 tablespoon lemon juice

- 1/4 teaspoon black pepper

- Whole grain crackers for serving

Nutritional facts (per serving):

- Calories: 150 kcal

- Protein: 1g

- Fat: 15g

- Carbohydrates: 5g

- Fiber: 2g

- Sodium: 600mg

Preparation directions:

1. In a food processor, combine the Kalamata olives, capers, garlic, parsley, olive oil, lemon juice, and black pepper.
2. Pulse until the mixture forms a coarse paste, scraping down the sides as needed.
3. Transfer the olive tapenade to a serving bowl.
4. Serve the tapenade with whole grain crackers for dipping or spreading.

Variations/Substitutions:

- Add a few anchovy fillets for a deeper umami flavor.
- Substitute lemon juice with balsamic vinegar for a sweeter taste.

Health Benefit:

Olive Tapenade on Whole Grain Crackers is a flavorful and heart-healthy snack that's perfect for a low sodium Mediterranean diet. Olives and olive oil are rich in monounsaturated fats, which can help reduce the risk of heart disease. The whole grain crackers provide a good source of fiber, supporting digestive health. This snack is a great way to enjoy a tasty and nutritious treat that aligns with the principles of a low sodium diet.

34. Stuffed Grape Leaves (Dolmas)

- Prep time: 30 minutes

- Cook time: 40 minutes

- Serving size: 4 servings (about 5 dolmas per serving)

Ingredients:

- 20 grape leaves, rinsed and drained

- 1 cup cooked brown rice

- 1/2 cup chopped fresh parsley

- 1/4 cup chopped fresh dill

- 1/4 cup chopped fresh mint

- 1/4 cup pine nuts

- 2 tablespoons olive oil

- 2 tablespoons lemon juice

- 1/4 teaspoon black pepper

- Lemon slices for garnish

Nutritional facts (per serving):

- Calories: 200 kcal

- Protein: 4g

- Fat: 10g

- Carbohydrates: 26g

- Fiber: 3g

- Sodium: 200mg

Preparation directions:

1. In a bowl, mix together the cooked brown rice, chopped parsley, dill, mint, pine nuts, 1 tablespoon of olive oil, lemon juice, and black pepper.
2. Lay a grape leaf flat on a work surface, vein side up. Place a spoonful of the rice mixture near the stem end of the leaf.
3. Fold in the sides of the leaf and roll it up tightly, starting from the stem end. Repeat with the remaining grape leaves and filling.
4. Arrange the stuffed grape leaves in a single layer in a large pot. Drizzle the remaining olive oil over the top.
5. Pour enough water into the pot to just cover the grape leaves. Place a plate on top to keep them submerged.
6. Bring the water to a boil, then reduce the heat and simmer for 40 minutes.
7. Remove the grape leaves from the pot and let them cool. Serve the dolmas with lemon slices.

Variations/Substitutions:

- Add cooked lentils or chickpeas to the filling for added protein.
- Substitute pine nuts with chopped almonds or walnuts for a different crunch.

Health Benefit:

Stuffed Grape Leaves (Dolmas) are a traditional Mediterranean snack that's both delicious and nutritious. The brown rice provides a good source of whole grains and fiber, while the fresh herbs add flavor and antioxidants. The olive oil contributes healthy fats, and the lemon juice adds a refreshing tang. These dolmas are a great option for a low sodium snack that's packed with wholesome ingredients.

35. Roasted Garlic and White Bean Dip

- Prep time: 10 minutes

- Cook time: 30 minutes

- Serving size: 4 servings

Ingredients:

- 1 head of garlic
- 1 tablespoon olive oil
- 1 can (15 oz) no-salt-added white beans (such as cannellini or navy beans), rinsed and drained
- 2 tablespoons lemon juice
- 2 tablespoons tahini
- 1/4 teaspoon black pepper
- Fresh parsley or rosemary for garnish
- Vegetable sticks or whole grain pita chips for serving

Nutritional facts (per serving):

- Calories: 150 kcal

- Protein: 7g

- Fat: 5g

- Carbohydrates: 20g

- Fiber: 5g

- Sodium: 15mg

Preparation directions:

1. Preheat the oven to 400°F (200°C).

2. Slice off the top of the garlic head to expose the cloves. Drizzle with olive oil and wrap in foil. Roast in the oven for 30 minutes, or until the cloves are soft and golden.

3. Squeeze the roasted garlic cloves out of their skins and into a food processor.

4. Add the white beans, lemon juice, tahini, and black pepper to the food processor. Blend until smooth and creamy.

5. Transfer the dip to a serving bowl and garnish with fresh parsley or rosemary.

6. Serve the Roasted Garlic and White Bean Dip with vegetable sticks or whole grain pita chips.

Variations/Substitutions:

- Add a pinch of smoked paprika or cumin for extra flavor.

- Substitute tahini with almond butter for a nutty twist.

Health Benefit:

Roasted Garlic and White Bean Dip is a flavorful and nutritious snack that's perfect for a low sodium Mediterranean diet. White beans are an excellent source of plant-based protein and fiber, which can help support digestive health and keep you feeling full. The roasted garlic adds a rich, savory flavor without the need for added salt, while the olive oil provides healthy fats. This dip is a great way to enjoy a tasty and heart-healthy snack that's low in sodium.

36. Baked Zucchini Fries

- Prep time: 10 minutes

- Cook time: 20 minutes

- Serving size: 4 servings

Ingredients:

- 2 medium zucchinis, cut into fry-shaped sticks

- 1/2 cup whole wheat breadcrumbs

- 1/4 cup grated Parmesan cheese

- 1 teaspoon dried oregano

- 1/4 teaspoon black pepper

- 2 egg whites, beaten

- Cooking spray

Nutritional facts (per serving):

- Calories: 90 kcal

- Protein: 6g

- Fat: 2g

- Carbohydrates: 12g

- Fiber: 2g

- Sodium: 150mg

Preparation directions:

1. Preheat the oven to 425°F (220°C). Line a baking sheet with parchment paper and lightly coat with cooking spray.

2. In a shallow dish, mix together the whole wheat breadcrumbs, grated Parmesan cheese, dried oregano, and black pepper.

3. Dip each zucchini stick into the beaten egg whites, then coat with the breadcrumb mixture. Place the coated zucchini fries on the prepared baking sheet.

4. Bake in the preheated oven for 20 minutes, or until the zucchini fries are golden and crispy.

5. Serve the Baked Zucchini Fries hot, with a side of marinara sauce or Greek yogurt for dipping.

Variations/Substitutions:

- Use almond meal or crushed nuts instead of breadcrumbs for a gluten-free option.

- Add a pinch of garlic powder or cayenne pepper to the breadcrumb mixture for extra flavor.

Health Benefit:

Baked Zucchini Fries are a healthy and delicious alternative to traditional French fries. Zucchini is low in calories and high in vitamins and antioxidants, making it a great choice for a low sodium Mediterranean diet. The whole wheat breadcrumbs and Parmesan cheese provide a crispy coating without the need for deep frying, while the egg whites help bind the coating to the zucchini. This snack is a tasty way to enjoy a serving of vegetables with a satisfying crunch.

37. Mediterranean Salsa with Pita Chips

- *Prep time: 15 minutes*
- *Cook time: 10 minutes (for pita chips)*
- *Serving size: 4 servings*

Ingredients:

- 1 cup diced tomatoes
- 1 cup diced cucumber
- 1/2 cup diced red onion
- 1/2 cup chopped Kalamata olives
- 1/4 cup chopped fresh parsley
- 2 tablespoons lemon juice
- 2 tablespoons olive oil
- 1/4 teaspoon black pepper
- 4 whole wheat pita bread rounds
- Cooking spray

Nutritional facts (per serving):

- Calories: 200 kcal
- Protein: 5g
- Fat: 10g
- Carbohydrates: 25g
- Fiber: 4g
- Sodium: 300mg

Preparation directions:

1. In a bowl, combine the diced tomatoes, cucumber, red onion, Kalamata olives, and chopped parsley.
2. In a small bowl, whisk together the lemon juice, olive oil, and black pepper to make the dressing.
3. Pour the dressing over the salsa mixture and toss gently to coat.
4. Preheat the oven to 375°F (190°C). Cut each pita bread round into 8 wedges and arrange them on a baking sheet. Lightly spray the pita wedges with cooking spray.
5. Bake the pita chips in the oven for 10 minutes, or until crispy and golden.
6. Serve the Mediterranean Salsa with the homemade pita chips.

Variations/Substitutions:

- Add crumbled feta cheese or chickpeas to the salsa for added protein.
- Substitute lemon juice with balsamic vinegar for a different flavor profile.

Health Benefit:

Mediterranean Salsa with Pita Chips is a light and flavorful snack that's perfect for a low sodium Mediterranean diet. The salsa is packed with fresh vegetables and herbs, providing vitamins, minerals, and antioxidants. The whole wheat pita chips offer a crunchy and satisfying alternative to traditional chips, with the added benefit of fiber. This snack is a great way to enjoy a variety of nutrient-dense ingredients in a tasty and low sodium way.

38. Caprese Salad Skewers

- *Prep time: 10 minutes*

- *Serving size: 4 servings (3 skewers per serving)*

Ingredients:

- 12 cherry tomatoes

- 12 small mozzarella balls (bocconcini)

- 12 fresh basil leaves

- 2 tablespoons balsamic glaze

- 1 tablespoon olive oil

- 1/4 teaspoon black pepper

- Wooden skewers

Nutritional facts (per serving):

- Calories: 150

- Protein: 8g

- Fat: 11g

- Carbohydrates: 5g

- Fiber: 1g

- Sodium: 35mg

Preparation directions:

1. Assemble the skewers by threading a cherry tomato, a basil leaf, and a mozzarella ball onto each skewer. Repeat until all ingredients are used.
2. Arrange the skewers on a serving platter.
3. Drizzle the balsamic glaze and olive oil over the skewers.
4. Sprinkle with black pepper and serve.

Variations/Substitutions:

- Add a slice of cucumber or a piece of roasted red pepper between the tomato and mozzarella for added crunch and flavor.
- Substitute balsamic glaze with a squeeze of lemon juice for a citrusy twist.

Health Benefit:

Caprese Salad Skewers are a simple and elegant snack that's low in sodium and high in flavor. The cherry tomatoes and basil provide a good source of vitamins and antioxidants, while the mozzarella balls offer protein and calcium. The balsamic glaze and olive oil add a rich and tangy taste to the skewers, making them a delightful and nutritious option for a low sodium Mediterranean diet.

39. Artichoke and Spinach Dip

- *Prep time: 10 minutes*

- *Cook time: 25 minutes*

- *Serving size: 4 servings*

Ingredients:

- 1 can (14 oz) artichoke hearts, drained and chopped

- 2 cups fresh spinach, chopped

- 1/2 cup low-fat cream cheese, softened

- 1/4 cup plain Greek yogurt

- 1/4 cup grated Parmesan cheese

- 2 garlic cloves, minced

- 1/4 teaspoon black pepper

- Whole grain pita chips or vegetable sticks for serving

Nutritional facts (per serving):

- Calories: 150 kcal

- Protein: 8g

- Fat: 8g

- Carbohydrates: 12g

- Fiber: 3g

- Sodium: 300mg

Preparation directions:

1. Preheat the oven to 375°F (190°C).
2. In a bowl, mix together the chopped artichoke hearts, chopped spinach, cream cheese, Greek yogurt, Parmesan cheese, minced garlic, and black pepper.
3. Transfer the mixture to a baking dish and spread it evenly.
4. Bake in the preheated oven for 25 minutes, or until the dip is hot and bubbly.
5. Serve the Artichoke and Spinach Dip warm with whole grain pita chips or vegetable sticks for dipping.

Variations/Substitutions:

- Add a pinch of red pepper flakes for a spicy kick.
- Substitute Greek yogurt with low-fat sour cream for a different tangy flavor.

Health Benefit:

Artichoke and Spinach Dip is a creamy and delicious snack that's a great addition to a low sodium Mediterranean diet. Artichokes are a good source of fiber and antioxidants, while spinach provides vitamins A, C, and K, as well as iron. The combination of low-fat cream cheese and Greek yogurt adds protein and calcium without excessive sodium, making this dip a healthier alternative to traditional high-sodium versions.

40. Feta and Watermelon Bites

- Prep time: 10 minutes

- Serving size: 4 servings (3 bites per serving)

Ingredients:

- 12 small cubes of watermelon

- 12 small cubes of feta cheese

- 12 fresh mint leaves

- 1 tablespoon balsamic glaze

- Toothpicks

Nutritional facts (per serving):

- Calories: 70 kcal

- Protein: 3g

- Fat: 4g

- Carbohydrates: 6g

- Fiber: 0g

- Sodium: 200mg

Preparation directions:

1. Assemble the bites by placing a cube of watermelon on a toothpick, followed by a mint leaf and a cube of feta cheese.

2. Arrange the bites on a serving platter.

3. Drizzle the balsamic glaze over the bites just before serving.

Variations/Substitutions:

- Substitute watermelon with cantaloupe or honeydew melon for a different flavor.

- Use a squeeze of lime juice instead of balsamic glaze for a citrusy twist.

Health Benefit:

Feta and Watermelon Bites are a refreshing and light snack that's perfect for a low sodium Mediterranean diet. Watermelon is hydrating and rich in vitamins A and C, while feta cheese provides a salty contrast and a source of calcium. The mint adds a fresh flavor, and the balsamic glaze provides a sweet and tangy finish. These bites are a delightful way to enjoy a combination of flavors and nutrients in a low sodium, bite-sized treat.

41. Greek Yogurt with Honey and Walnuts

- Prep time: 5 minutes

- Serving size: 4 servings

Ingredients:

- 2 cups low-fat Greek yogurt

- 4 tablespoons honey

- 1/2 cup chopped walnuts

- 1/4 teaspoon ground cinnamon (optional)

Nutritional facts (per serving):

- Calories: 200 kcal

- Protein: 12g

- Fat: 10g

- Carbohydrates: 20g

- Fiber: 1g

- Sodium: 50mg

Preparation directions:

1. Divide the Greek yogurt evenly among four serving bowls.

2. Drizzle 1 tablespoon of honey over each serving of yogurt.

3. Sprinkle the chopped walnuts on top of the yogurt and honey.

4. If desired, add a pinch of ground cinnamon to each serving for added flavor.

5. Serve immediately and enjoy a simple and nutritious dessert.

Variations/Substitutions:

- Substitute walnuts with almonds or pistachios for a different nutty flavor.

- Add fresh berries or sliced fruit for added sweetness and vitamins.

Health Benefit:

Greek Yogurt with Honey and Walnuts is a healthy and satisfying dessert that's perfect for a low sodium Mediterranean diet. Greek yogurt provides a good source of protein and calcium, while the honey adds natural sweetness. Walnuts are rich in healthy fats and antioxidants, making this dessert a great choice for heart health. The combination of flavors and textures makes this a delightful way to end a meal or enjoy a snack.

42. Poached Pears in Red Wine

- *Prep time: 10 minutes*

- *Cook time: 30 minutes*

- *Serving size: 4 servings*

Ingredients:

- 4 ripe pears, peeled and cored

- 2 cups red wine

- 1/2 cup honey

- 1 cinnamon stick

- 1 strip of orange zest

- 1/4 teaspoon ground cloves

Nutritional facts (per serving):

- Calories: 280 kcal

- Protein: 1g

- Fat: 0g

- Carbohydrates: 50g

- Fiber: 4g

- Sodium: 10mg

Preparation directions:

1. In a large saucepan, combine the red wine, honey, cinnamon stick, orange zest, and ground cloves. Bring the mixture to a simmer over medium heat.
2. Add the peeled and cored pears to the saucepan, making sure they are submerged in the wine.
3. Simmer the pears for 30 minutes, turning them occasionally, until they are tender and have absorbed the color of the wine.
4. Carefully remove the pears from the saucepan and place them in serving dishes.
5. Continue simmering the wine sauce until it reduces to a syrupy consistency.
6. Pour the reduced wine sauce over the pears and serve.

Variations/Substitutions:

- Substitute red wine with white wine or apple juice for a different flavor profile.
- Add a vanilla pod to the poaching liquid for added sweetness and aroma.

Health Benefit:

Poached Pears in Red Wine is a sophisticated and healthy dessert that's low in sodium and rich in flavor. Pears are a good source of fiber and antioxidants, while the red wine and spices add depth and complexity to the dish. This dessert is a great way to enjoy the natural sweetness of fruit with the added benefits of heart-healthy polyphenols from the wine.

43. Fig and Almond Cake

- *Prep time: 15 minutes*
- *Cook time: 30 minutes*
- *Serving size: 8 servings*

Ingredients:

- 1 cup almond flour

- 1/2 cup whole wheat flour

- 1/2 cup honey

- 1/4 cup olive oil

- 3 large eggs

- 1 teaspoon baking powder

- 1/4 teaspoon salt

- 1 teaspoon vanilla extract

- 1 cup chopped dried figs

- 1/4 cup sliced almonds

Nutritional facts (per serving):

- Calories: 280 kcal

- Protein: 7g

- Fat: 15g

- Carbohydrates: 32g

- Fiber: 4g

- Sodium: 100mg

Preparation directions:

1. Preheat the oven to 350°F (175°C). Grease and flour an 8-inch cake pan.

2. In a large bowl, mix together the almond flour, whole wheat flour, baking powder, and salt.

3. In a separate bowl, whisk together the honey, olive oil, eggs, and vanilla extract.

4. Gradually add the wet ingredients to the dry ingredients, stirring until well combined.

5. Fold in the chopped dried figs.

6. Pour the batter into the prepared cake pan and smooth the top with a spatula.

7. Sprinkle the sliced almonds over the top of the batter.

8. Bake in the preheated oven for 30 minutes, or until a toothpick inserted into the center of the cake comes out clean.

9. Let the cake cool in the pan for 10 minutes, then transfer to a wire rack to cool completely.

Variations/Substitutions:

- Substitute honey with maple syrup for a different sweetness.

- Add a teaspoon of ground cinnamon or cardamom for added spice.

Health Benefit:

Fig and Almond Cake is a delightful dessert that's perfect for a low sodium Mediterranean diet. Almond flour provides a good source of protein and healthy fats, while whole wheat flour adds fiber. Figs are rich in vitamins, minerals, and antioxidants, making this cake a healthier option compared to traditional sugary desserts. The use of honey and olive oil instead of refined sugar and butter makes this cake a heart-healthy choice that's lower in sodium and added sugars.

44. Orange and Almond Biscotti

- *Prep time: 20 minutes*

- *Cook time: 40 minutes*

- *Serving size: 16 biscotti*

Ingredients:

- 2 cups almond flour

- 1/2 cup whole wheat flour

- 1/2 cup honey

- 2 large eggs

- 1 tablespoon orange zest

- 1 teaspoon vanilla extract

- 1/2 teaspoon baking powder

- 1/4 teaspoon salt

- 1/4 cup sliced almonds

Nutritional facts (per biscotti):

- Calories: 150 kcal

- Protein: 5g

- Fat: 10g

- Carbohydrates: 12g

- Fiber: 2g

- Sodium: 40mg

Preparation directions:

1. Preheat the oven to 350°F (175°C). Line a baking sheet with parchment paper.
2. In a large bowl, mix together the almond flour, whole wheat flour, baking powder, and salt.
3. In a separate bowl, whisk together the honey, eggs, orange zest, and vanilla extract.
4. Gradually add the wet ingredients to the dry ingredients, stirring until well combined.
5. Form the dough into a log shape on the prepared baking sheet. Flatten the log slightly so it's about 1 inch thick.
6. Sprinkle the sliced almonds over the top of the dough.
7. Bake in the preheated oven for 25 minutes, or until the log is lightly golden and firm to the touch.
8. Remove from the oven and let cool for 10 minutes. Reduce the oven temperature to 300°F (150°C).
9. Using a serrated knife, slice the log diagonally into 1/2-inch thick biscotti.
10. Arrange the biscotti cut-side down on the baking sheet and bake for an additional 15 minutes, or until crisp and golden.
11. Let the biscotti cool completely on a wire rack.

Variations/Substitutions:

- Substitute orange zest with lemon zest for a different citrus flavor.

- Add a teaspoon of ground cinnamon or nutmeg for added warmth.

Health Benefit:

Orange and Almond Biscotti are a delightful and healthy treat that's perfect for a low sodium Mediterranean diet. Almond flour provides a good source of protein and healthy fats, while the orange zest adds a refreshing citrus flavor and vitamin C. These biscotti are a great alternative to traditional high-sugar, high-sodium desserts, offering a satisfying crunch and natural sweetness from honey.

45. Lemon and Olive Oil Cake

- Prep time: 15 minutes

- Cook time: 35 minutes

- Serving size: 8 servings

Ingredients:

- 1 1/2 cups whole wheat flour

- 1/2 cup almond flour

- 3/4 cup honey

- 1/2 cup olive oil

- 3 large eggs

- 2 tablespoons lemon zest

- 1/4 cup fresh lemon juice

- 1 teaspoon baking powder

- 1/4 teaspoon salt

- Powdered sugar for dusting (optional)

Nutritional facts (per serving):

- Calories: 320 kcal

- Protein: 6g

- Fat: 18g

- Carbohydrates: 36g

- Fiber: 3g

- Sodium: 90mg

Preparation directions:

1. Preheat the oven to 350°F (175°C). Grease and flour a 9-inch cake pan.

2. In a large bowl, mix together the whole wheat flour, almond flour, baking powder, and salt.

3. In a separate bowl, whisk together the honey, olive oil, eggs, lemon zest, and lemon juice.

4. Gradually add the wet ingredients to the dry ingredients, stirring until well combined.

5. Pour the batter into the prepared cake pan and smooth the top with a spatula.

6. Bake in the preheated oven for 35 minutes, or until a toothpick inserted into the center of the cake comes out clean.

7. Let the cake cool in the pan for 10 minutes, then transfer to a wire rack to cool completely.

8. If desired, dust the top of the cake with powdered sugar before serving.

Variations/Substitutions:

- Substitute honey with maple syrup for a different sweetness.
- Add a tablespoon of poppy seeds to the batter for added texture.

Health Benefit:

Lemon and Olive Oil Cake is a moist and flavorful dessert that's perfect for a low sodium Mediterranean diet. Olive oil provides heart-healthy monounsaturated fats, while the lemon adds a refreshing burst of flavor and vitamin C. Whole wheat and almond flours offer a good source of fiber and nutrients, making this cake a healthier option compared to traditional cakes made with refined flours and sugars.

46. Baklava with Pistachios

- *Prep time: 20 minutes*

- *Cook time: 45 minutes*

- *Serving size: 12 servings*

Ingredients:

- 1 package phyllo dough, thawed

- 2 cups chopped pistachios

- 1/2 cup honey

- 1/2 cup water

- 1/4 cup olive oil

- 1 teaspoon ground cinnamon

- 1/4 teaspoon ground cloves

Nutritional facts (per serving):

- Calories: 280 kcal

- Protein: 5g

- Fat: 15g

- Carbohydrates: 32g

- Fiber: 2g

- Sodium: 120mg

Preparation directions:

1. Preheat the oven to 350°F (175°C). Grease a 9x13-inch baking dish.
2. In a bowl, mix together the chopped pistachios, cinnamon, and ground cloves.
3. Lay one sheet of phyllo dough in the prepared baking dish and brush with olive oil. Repeat with 4 more sheets, brushing each with oil.
4. Sprinkle a layer of the pistachio mixture over the phyllo. Add another 5 layers of phyllo, brushing each with oil.
5. Continue layering the phyllo and pistachio mixture until all ingredients are used, finishing with a layer of phyllo on top.
6. Using a sharp knife, cut the baklava into diamond-shaped pieces.
7. Bake in the preheated oven for 45 minutes, or until golden and crisp.
8. While the baklava is baking, heat the honey and water in a saucepan over medium heat until the honey is dissolved. Simmer for 5 minutes.
9. Pour the warm honey syrup over the hot baklava as soon as it comes out of the oven.
10. Let the baklava cool completely before serving.

Variations/Substitutions:

- Substitute pistachios with walnuts or almonds for a different flavor.
- Add a tablespoon of orange zest to the honey syrup for a citrusy twist.

Health Benefit:

Baklava with Pistachios is a classic Mediterranean dessert that's rich in flavor and texture. Pistachios provide healthy fats, protein, and antioxidants, while the honey adds natural sweetness without the need for refined sugars. While baklava is a treat best enjoyed in moderation, this version uses olive oil instead of butter, making it a slightly healthier option that still adheres to the principles of a low sodium Mediterranean diet.

47. Ricotta and Lemon Zest Crepes

- Prep time: 15 minutes

- Cook time: 20 minutes

- Serving size: 4 servings (2 crepes per serving)

Ingredients:

- 1 cup whole wheat flour
- 1 1/2 cups low-fat milk
- 2 large eggs

- 1 tablespoon olive oil

- 1/2 teaspoon salt

- Cooking spray

- 1 cup low-fat ricotta cheese

- 2 tablespoons honey

- 1 tablespoon lemon zest

- Powdered sugar for dusting (optional)

Nutritional facts (per serving):

- Calories: 320 kcal

- Protein: 16g

- Fat: 12g

- Carbohydrates: 38g

- Fiber: 4g

- Sodium: 380mg

Preparation directions:

1. In a blender, combine the whole wheat flour, milk, eggs, olive oil, and salt. Blend until smooth to create the crepe batter.

2. Heat a non-stick skillet over medium heat and lightly coat with cooking spray.

3. Pour 1/4 cup of the crepe batter into the skillet, tilting to spread evenly. Cook for 2 minutes, or until the edges start

to lift. Flip and cook for another 1-2 minutes. Repeat with the remaining batter.

4. In a bowl, mix together the ricotta cheese, honey, and lemon zest.

5. Spread the ricotta mixture over each crepe and roll them up.

6. Serve the crepes dusted with powdered sugar, if desired.

Variations/Substitutions:

- Substitute whole wheat flour with almond flour for a gluten-free option.

- Add fresh berries or sliced fruit on top of the ricotta filling for added sweetness and vitamins.

Health Benefit:

Ricotta and Lemon Zest Crepes are a light and delicious dessert that's suitable for a low sodium Mediterranean diet. The whole wheat crepes provide a good source of fiber, while the ricotta cheese adds protein and calcium. The lemon zest adds a refreshing citrus flavor and a boost of vitamin C. This dessert is a great way to enjoy a sweet treat that's lower in sodium and made with wholesome ingredients.

48. Chocolate-Dipped Dried Fruits

- *Prep time: 15 minutes*

- *Chill time: 30 minutes*

- *Serving size: 4 servings*

Ingredients:

- 1/2 cup dark chocolate chips (70% cocoa or higher)

- 1 cup mixed dried fruits (such as apricots, figs, and dates)

- 1/4 cup chopped nuts (such as almonds or pistachios)

Nutritional facts (per serving):

- Calories: 220 kcal

- Protein: 3g

- Fat: 10g

- Carbohydrates: 32g

- Fiber: 4g

- Sodium: 20mg

Preparation directions:

1. Melt the dark chocolate chips in a heatproof bowl set over a pot of simmering water, stirring until smooth.

2. Dip half of each piece of dried fruit into the melted chocolate, then place them on a parchment-lined baking sheet.

3. Sprinkle the chopped nuts over the chocolate-covered portion of the fruit.

4. Place the baking sheet in the refrigerator and chill for 30 minutes, or until the chocolate is set.

5. Serve the chocolate-dipped dried fruits as a sweet and nutritious snack.

Variations/Substitutions:

- Use white or milk chocolate for a different flavor, though this will increase the sugar content.

- Roll the chocolate-dipped fruits in shredded coconut or cocoa powder instead of nuts.

Health Benefit:

Chocolate-Dipped Dried Fruits are a simple and elegant dessert that's perfect for a low sodium Mediterranean diet. Dark chocolate is rich in antioxidants and can have heart-healthy benefits when consumed in moderation. Dried fruits provide natural sweetness and are a good source of fiber and vitamins. The addition of nuts adds healthy fats and a crunchy texture, making this a balanced and indulgent treat.

49. Honey and Sesame Seed Bars

- *Prep time: 10 minutes*

- *Cook time: 20 minutes*

- *Chill time: 30 minutes*

- *Serving size: 8 bars*

Ingredients:

- 1 cup rolled oats

- 1/2 cup sesame seeds

- 1/2 cup chopped almonds

- 1/4 cup honey

- 1/4 cup almond butter

- 1 teaspoon vanilla extract

- 1/4 teaspoon salt

Nutritional facts (per bar):

- Calories: 180 kcal

- Protein: 5g

- Fat: 11g

- Carbohydrates: 16g

- Fiber: 3g

- Sodium: 75mg

Preparation directions:

1. Preheat the oven to 350°F (175°C). Line an 8x8-inch baking dish with parchment paper.
2. In a large bowl, mix together the rolled oats, sesame seeds, and chopped almonds.
3. In a small saucepan, heat the honey and almond butter over low heat until melted and smooth. Stir in the vanilla extract and salt.
4. Pour the honey mixture over the oat mixture and stir until well combined.
5. Press the mixture firmly into the prepared baking dish.
6. Bake in the preheated oven for 20 minutes, or until the edges are golden brown.
7. Let the bars cool in the dish for 10 minutes, then transfer to the refrigerator to chill for 30 minutes.
8. Cut into bars and serve.

Variations/Substitutions:

- Substitute almond butter with peanut butter or tahini for a different flavor.
- Add dried fruits, such as cranberries or raisins, for added sweetness and texture.

Health Benefit:

Honey and Sesame Seed Bars are a wholesome and satisfying snack that's ideal for a low sodium Mediterranean diet. The rolled oats provide a good source of fiber, while the sesame seeds and almonds offer healthy fats, protein, and minerals. The honey adds natural sweetness without the need for refined sugars. These bars are a great way to enjoy a nutritious and portable snack that's lower in sodium and packed with flavor.

50. Pomegranate and Yogurt Parfait

- Prep time: 10 minutes

- Serving size: 4 servings

Ingredients:

- 2 cups low-fat Greek yogurt

- 1 cup pomegranate seeds

- 1/4 cup honey

- 1/4 cup granola

- 1 teaspoon ground cinnamon

Nutritional facts (per serving):

- Calories: 200 kcal

- Protein: 12g

- Fat: 3g

- Carbohydrates: 34g

- Fiber: 3g

- Sodium: 60mg

Preparation directions:

1. In a serving glass or bowl, layer 1/4 cup of Greek yogurt.
2. Sprinkle a layer of pomegranate seeds over the yogurt.
3. Drizzle 1 tablespoon of honey over the pomegranate seeds.
4. Add another layer of Greek yogurt, followed by a layer of granola.
5. Repeat the layers until all ingredients are used, finishing with a layer of pomegranate seeds on top.
6. Sprinkle ground cinnamon over the parfait before serving.

Variations/Substitutions:

- Substitute pomegranate seeds with mixed berries or sliced fruit for a different flavor.
- Use agave syrup or maple syrup instead of honey for a vegan option.

Health Benefit:

Pomegranate and Yogurt Parfait is a refreshing and nutritious dessert that's perfect for a low sodium Mediterranean diet. Greek yogurt provides a rich source of protein and probiotics, supporting digestive health. Pomegranate seeds are packed with antioxidants and vitamins, while the granola adds a satisfying crunch. This parfait is a delightful way to enjoy a balanced and flavorful treat that's low in sodium and high in nutrients.

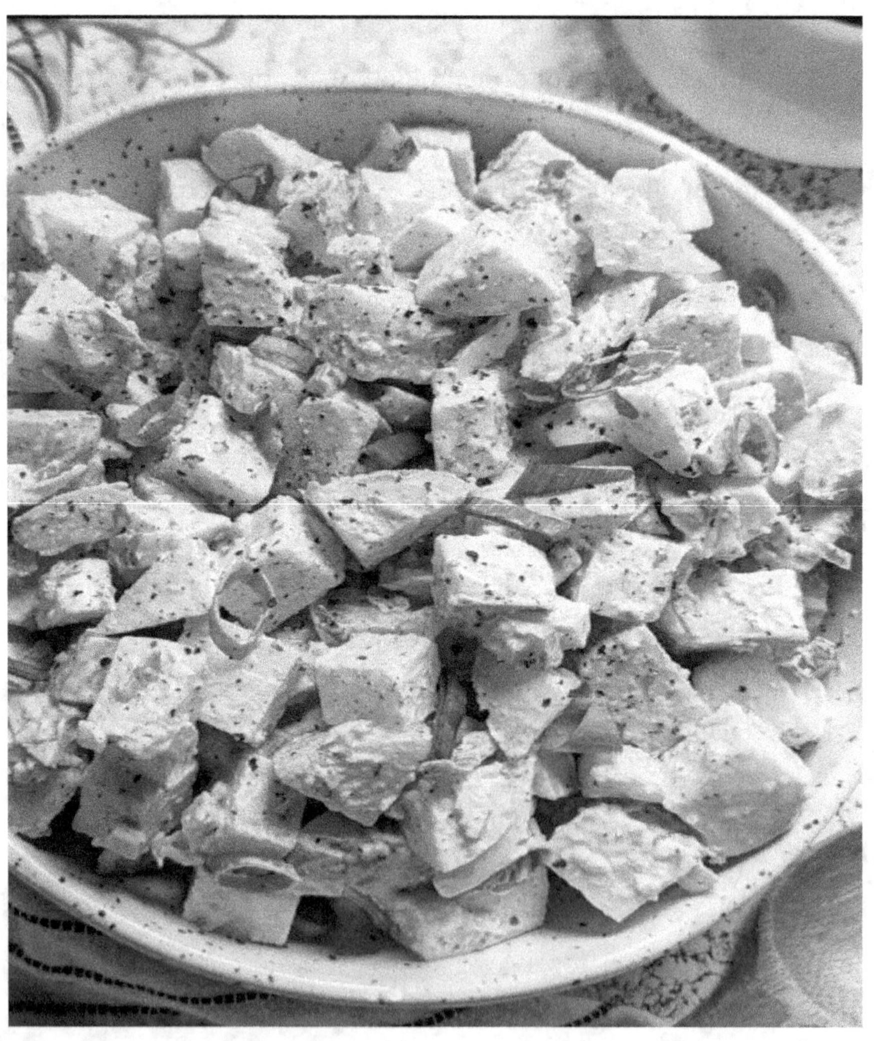

6. 14-DAY LOW SODIUM MEDITERRANEAN MEAL PLAN

Day 1

- Breakfast: Greek Yogurt with Honey and Walnuts (Recipe 41)

- Lunch: Mediterranean Chickpea Salad (Recipe 17)

- Snack: Hummus with Roasted Vegetables (Recipe 31)

- Dinner: Grilled Salmon with Lemon and Herbs (Recipe 21) and Quinoa Tabbouleh Salad (Recipe 13)

Day 2

- Breakfast: Lemon Ricotta Pancakes (Recipe 6)

- Lunch: Stuffed Bell Peppers with Quinoa (Recipe 24)

- Snack: Tzatziki with Cucumber Slices (Recipe 32)

- Dinner: Vegetable Paella (Recipe 22) with a side of Caprese Salad Skewers (Recipe 38)

- Breakfast: Mediterranean Breakfast Quinoa (Recipe 7)

- Lunch: White Bean and Arugula Salad (Recipe 15)

- Snack: Olive Tapenade on Whole Grain Crackers (Recipe 33)

- Dinner: Baked Chicken with Olives and Tomatoes (Recipe 23) and Roasted Garlic and White Bean Dip (Recipe 35) with vegetable sticks

- Breakfast: Almond and Date Overnight Oats (Recipe 8)

- Lunch: Greek Salad with Lemon Dressing (Recipe 11)

- Snack: Feta and Watermelon Bites (Recipe 40)

- Dinner: Lemon and Herb Baked Cod (Recipe 27) with a side of Mediterranean Salsa with Pita Chips (Recipe 37)

Day 5

- Breakfast: Shakshuka with Feta (Recipe 9)

- Lunch: Eggplant and Tomato Salad (Recipe 18)

- Snack: Baked Zucchini Fries (Recipe 36) with a side of Greek Yogurt

- Dinner: Eggplant Moussaka (Recipe 25) with a side of Artichoke and Spinach Dip (Recipe 39) and whole grain pita chips

---

Day 6

- Breakfast: Cucumber and Yogurt Smoothie (Recipe 10)

- Lunch: Lentil and Vegetable Soup (Recipe 12) with a side of whole grain bread

- Snack: Ricotta and Lemon Zest Crepes (Recipe 47)

- Dinner: Mediterranean Vegetable Stew (Recipe 26) with a side of whole grain bread

---

Day 7

- Breakfast: Avocado and Egg Breakfast Bowl (Recipe 5)

- Lunch: Tomato and Cucumber Gazpacho (Recipe 14) with whole grain crackers

- Snack: Chocolate-Dipped Dried Fruits (Recipe 48)

- Dinner: Spinach and Feta Stuffed Chicken (Recipe 28) with a side of roasted vegetables

---

Day 8

- Breakfast: Olive and Tomato Breakfast Toast (Recipe 3)

- Lunch: Roasted Red Pepper and Almond Soup (Recipe 16) with whole grain bread

- Snack: Honey and Sesame Seed Bars (Recipe 49)

- Dinner: Ratatouille with Herbed Couscous (Recipe 29) with a side of mixed greens

Day 9

- Breakfast: Lemon Ricotta Pancakes (Recipe 6)

- Lunch: Stuffed Grape Leaves (Dolmas) (Recipe 34) with a side of Greek yogurt

- Snack: Hummus with Roasted Vegetables (Recipe 31)

- Dinner: Grilled Vegetable and Halloumi Skewers (Recipe 30) with a side of whole grain pita bread

Day 10

- Breakfast: Mediterranean Breakfast Quinoa (Recipe 7)

- Lunch: White Bean and Arugula Salad (Recipe 15) with whole grain bread

- Snack: Tzatziki with Cucumber Slices (Recipe 32)

- Dinner: Baked Chicken with Olives and Tomatoes (Recipe 23) with a side of Quinoa Tabbouleh Salad (Recipe 13)

- Breakfast: Shakshuka with Feta (Recipe 9)

- Lunch: Greek Salad with Lemon Dressing (Recipe 11) with whole grain pita bread

- Snack: Olive Tapenade on Whole Grain Crackers (Recipe 33)

- Dinner: Vegetable Paella (Recipe 22) with a side of Caprese Salad Skewers (Recipe 38)

Day 12

- Breakfast: Almond and Date Overnight Oats (Recipe 8)

- Lunch: Eggplant and Tomato Salad (Recipe 18) with whole grain bread

- Snack: Feta and Watermelon Bites (Recipe 40)

- Dinner: Lemon and Herb Baked Cod (Recipe 27) with a side of Mediterranean Salsa with Pita Chips (Recipe 37)

- Breakfast: Cucumber and Yogurt Smoothie (Recipe 10)
- Lunch: Lentil and Vegetable Soup (Recipe 12) with a side of whole grain bread
- Snack: Ricotta and Lemon Zest Crepes (Recipe 47)
- Dinner: Eggplant Moussaka (Recipe 25) with a side of Artichoke and Spinach Dip (Recipe 39) and whole grain pita chips

Day 14

- Breakfast: Olive and Tomato Breakfast Toast (Recipe 3)
- Lunch: Tomato and Cucumber Gazpacho (Recipe 14) with whole grain crackers
- Snack: Baked Zucchini Fries (Recipe 36) with a side of Greek Yogurt
- Dinner: Mediterranean Vegetable Stew (Recipe 26) with a side of whole grain bread

Feel free to mix and match the meals based on your preferences and dietary needs. This meal plan provides a variety of flavors and nutrients to help you enjoy a low sodium Mediterranean diet.

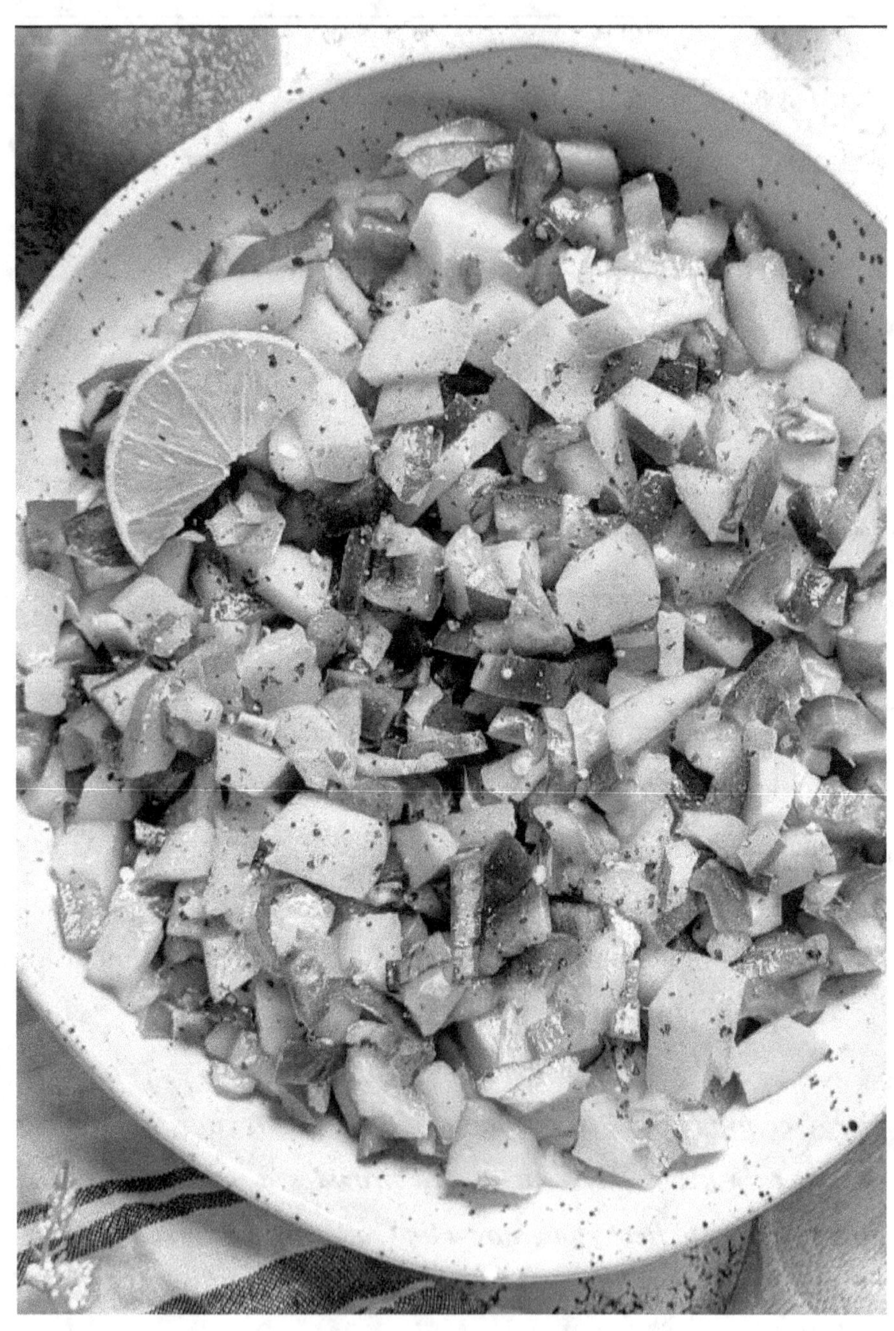

7. LIVING THE LOW SODIUM MEDITERRANEAN LIFESTYLE

Tips for Dining Out and Social Gatherings

When adopting a low sodium Mediterranean lifestyle, dining out and attending social gatherings can present challenges. However, with some planning and smart choices, you can enjoy these occasions without compromising your dietary goals.

1. Research Restaurants: Before dining out, research restaurants that offer Mediterranean or health-conscious options. Many establishments provide menus online, allowing you to review their offerings and identify suitable dishes.

2. Communicate with the Staff: When ordering, don't hesitate to ask questions about how the food is prepared. Request that your dish be prepared with less salt or no added salt. Most chefs are accommodating and can modify dishes to meet your needs.

3. Choose Wisely: Opt for grilled, baked, or steamed dishes over fried ones. Select lean proteins like fish, chicken, or legumes, and pair them with a side of vegetables or a salad. Avoid dishes with heavy sauces, as they often contain high levels of sodium.

4. Watch Portion Sizes: Restaurant portions can be generous. Consider sharing a dish with a friend or asking for a half portion. This not only helps control sodium intake but also prevents overeating.

5. Be Mindful of Appetizers and Sides: Opt for a salad with olive oil and vinegar dressing or a vegetable-based appetizer. Avoid bread baskets, salty snacks, and creamy dips, which can quickly add up in sodium content.

6. Stay Hydrated: Choose water or unsweetened beverages over sugary drinks or alcoholic beverages, which can contribute to dehydration and increased sodium retention.

7. Navigating Social Gatherings: At parties or social events, focus on fresh fruits, vegetables, nuts, and whole grains. If you're bringing a dish, prepare a low sodium Mediterranean option, such as a quinoa salad or a fruit platter, to ensure there's a healthy choice available.

8. *Practice Moderation:* It's okay to indulge occasionally, but be mindful of portion sizes and make balanced choices. Enjoying a small amount of a higher sodium dish can be part of a healthy lifestyle when balanced with other low sodium options.

By following these tips, you can confidently navigate dining out and social gatherings while maintaining a low sodium Mediterranean lifestyle. Making informed choices and communicating your dietary needs can help you enjoy a variety of foods and social experiences without compromising your health goals.

Incorporating Physical Activity and Mindfulness

Embracing a low sodium Mediterranean lifestyle involves more than just dietary changes; it also includes incorporating regular physical activity and mindfulness practices. These elements are crucial for overall well-being and complement the nutritional aspects of the Mediterranean diet.

1. *Regular Physical Activity:* Aim for at least 150 minutes of moderate aerobic activity or 75 minutes of vigorous activity each week, as recommended by the World Health Organization. This can include walking, jogging, cycling, swimming, or any other activity that gets your heart rate up. Additionally, incorporate strength training exercises at least two days a week to maintain muscle mass and bone health.

2. *Choose Activities You Enjoy:* The key to maintaining an active lifestyle is to find activities that you enjoy and look forward to. Whether it's dancing, hiking, yoga, or team sports, choose exercises that bring you joy and fit into your lifestyle.

3. *Incorporate Movement into Daily Life:* Beyond structured exercise, look for opportunities to move more throughout the day. Take the stairs instead of the elevator, go for a walk during your lunch break, or do some stretching while watching TV. Every bit of movement counts towards your overall activity level.

4. *Mindfulness and Stress Management:* Mindfulness practices, such as meditation, deep breathing, or progressive muscle relaxation, can help reduce stress and improve mental well-being. Set aside time each day to focus on your breath, observe your thoughts without judgment, and bring your attention to the present moment.

5. Connect with Nature: Spending time in nature has been shown to reduce stress, improve mood, and enhance physical health. Take walks in a park, garden, or by the sea to connect with the natural world and enjoy the calming effects of nature.

6. Practice Gratitude: Cultivate a sense of gratitude by taking time each day to reflect on the things you are thankful for. This can help shift your focus from what's lacking to what's abundant in your life, promoting a positive mindset.

7. Get Adequate Sleep: Quality sleep is essential for overall health and well-being. Aim for 7-9 hours of sleep per night, and establish a regular sleep routine to support your body's natural sleep-wake cycle.

8. Stay Connected: Social connections are an important aspect of the Mediterranean lifestyle. Spend time with family and friends, share meals, and engage in community activities to foster a sense of belonging and support.

By integrating physical activity and mindfulness practices into your daily routine, you can enhance the benefits of the low sodium Mediterranean diet and promote a holistic approach to health and well-being.

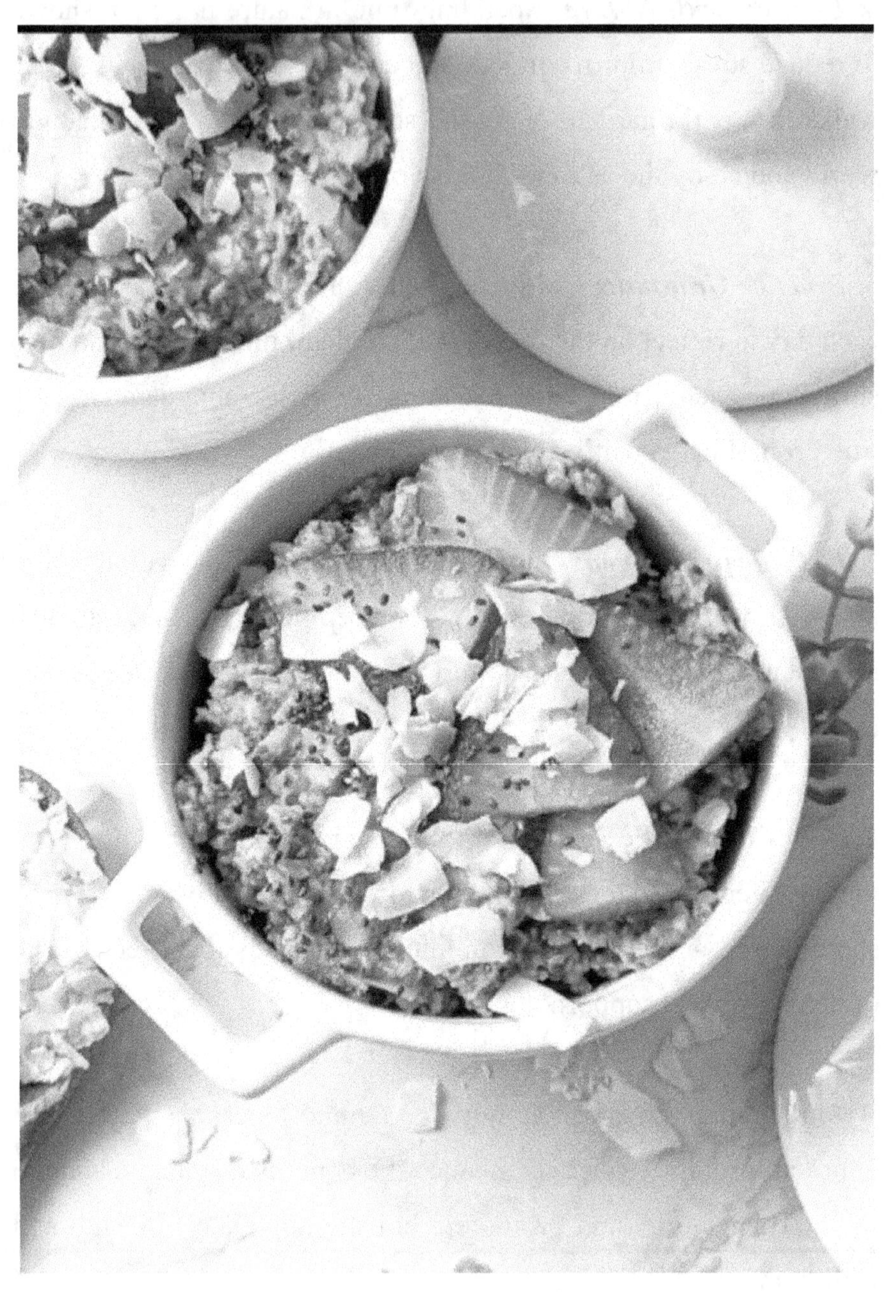

CONCLUSION

Encouragement and Final Thoughts for a Healthier Journey

As you embark on your journey toward a low sodium Mediterranean lifestyle, it's important to remember that this is not just a diet, but a holistic approach to living that encompasses nutrition, physical activity, mindfulness, and social connections. Embracing this lifestyle can lead to numerous health benefits, including improved heart health, better blood pressure control, and enhanced overall well-being.

Here are some final thoughts and words of encouragement:

1. Be Patient and Kind to Yourself: Changing habits takes time and effort. Be patient with yourself and celebrate small victories along the way. Remember that progress is not always linear, and it's okay to have setbacks. What's important is that you keep moving forward.

2. Focus on the Journey, Not Just the Destination: Enjoy the process of discovering new foods, recipes, and activities. The Mediterranean lifestyle is about savoring life and finding joy in the simple pleasures.

3. Listen to Your Body: Pay attention to how your body responds to different foods and activities. Use this feedback to adjust your choices and find what works best for you.

4. Seek Support: Share your journey with friends, family, or a support group. Having a support system can provide motivation, accountability, and encouragement when you need it most.

5. Embrace Flexibility: Life is unpredictable, and flexibility is key to maintaining a balanced lifestyle. Be open to adapting your plans and finding creative solutions to stay on track.

6. Prioritize Self-Care: Taking care of your physical, mental, and emotional health is essential. Make self-care a priority, and remember that taking time for yourself is not selfish, but necessary for your well-being.

7. *Stay Informed:* Continue to educate yourself about nutrition, physical activity, and mindfulness. The more you know, the better equipped you'll be to make informed decisions about your health.

As you move forward, remember that the low sodium Mediterranean lifestyle is not just about what you eat, but how you live. It's about finding balance, enjoying life, and nurturing your body, mind, and spirit. Here's to a healthier, happier, and more vibrant journey ahead!

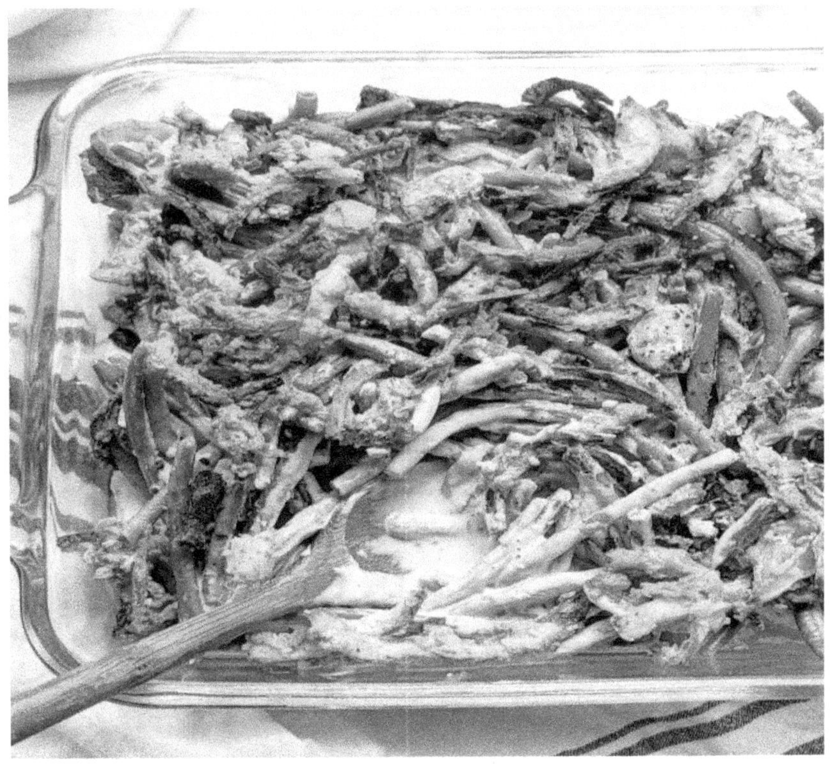